HERBAL REMEDIES FROM
THE WILD

HERBAL REMEDIES FROM
THE WILD

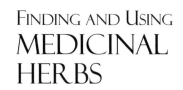

FINDING AND USING
MEDICINAL
HERBS

Corinne Martin
Illustrations by Helen Taylor

THE COUNTRYMAN PRESS
WOODSTOCK, VERMONT

Library of Congress Cataloging-in-Publication Data
Martin, Corinne, 1947–
    [Earthmagic]
    Herbal remedies from the wild : finding and using medicinal herbs / by
Corinne Martin ; illustrations by Helen Taylor.
        p. cm.
    Includes bibliographic references and index.
    ISBN 0-88150-485-8 (alk. paper)
        1. Herbs—Therapeutic use. 2. Herbals. I. Title.
RM666.H33 M373 2000
615'.321—dc21
                                            00-063847

Originally published by The Countryman Press in 1991 as *Earthmagic:
    Finding and Using Medicinal Herbs*
Copyright © 1991, 2000 by Corinne Martin

COVER AND INTERIOR DESIGN BY DEDE CUMMINGS DESIGNS
Cover photograph © Photodisc
Illustrations by Helen Taylor

Published by The Countryman Press
P.O. Box 748
Woodstock, Vermont 05091
A division of W.W. Norton & Co., Inc.
500 Fifth Avenue, New York, NY 10110

Printed in the United States of America
10 9 8 7 6 5 4 3 2 1

CONTENTS

DEDICATION

To my father—
>   *for country walks, for rides down the bayou, for trips to
>   Grandma's house, for strength and safety, for all the work, and
>   in the end, for dignity.*

And to my mother—
>   *for rescued baby birds, for fun and laughter, for the garden and
>   the animals, for affection, and for the joy of everyday things.*

ACKNOWLEDGMENTS

This book would not be complete without acknowledging those who helped make it possible. Many thanks to Helen Taylor for stopping in the middle of everything to draw the dirty, ragged plant that needed to be captured right away, and for planting it when the work was done. Thanks also to: Rosemary Gladstar, for reviewing the material and making helpful suggestions; my daughters Lara and Alison for being willing to try whatever I brewed up; and Minerva Martin, for help with herb school. Special thanks to Cathy Grigsby and Cathy DeLauter for always being there for me in one way or another, and to Bev for restoring me in the first place.

NOTICE TO THE READER

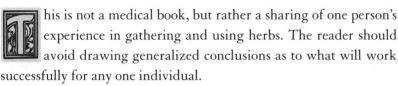his is not a medical book, but rather a sharing of one person's experience in gathering and using herbs. The reader should avoid drawing generalized conclusions as to what will work successfully for any one individual.

The simple herbal medicines discussed in this book are only one aspect of a medical care program. Any serious illness or warning symptom calls for diagnosis and treatment by a qualified physician.

Remember, each individual is different and will respond uniquely to herbal treatments. Not all applications are effective in every case for every person. Use herbs with care and moderation, keeping track of individual responses to carefully limited applications.

If you are sensitive to many substances, try only one herb at a time in small dosages, and then record any side effects. If none is present, increase the dosage or frequency *cautiously* and on a limited basis and continue to monitor for any adverse reaction. Take the same precautions with herbal medicines that you would with other medicines in your home. Label all containers.

PREFACE

Mid-December, early morning. A fierce wind has blown all night. This morning the house still shivers and windows make a popping sound with every furious gust. Tiny snowflakes have gotten bigger in the past hour, but the sky is still dark and the mountain beyond the field has disappeared. The bird feeder flaps crazily in the wind. So far no birds have braved the morning cold for seed.

Out the back window, the fields look like a vast white desert. Wind sweeps across the snow, sucking it up into tall plumes that twist and lift and dance along the ground until they disappear. I have sat at the kitchen table for half an hour, watching the wind and snow as the sky lightened into a paler shade of gray, and still I can't stop watching. In front of the house the plow has come once already, sweeping snow into great walls that make the road a white tunnel, but minutes later new drifts formed and again the road is gone.

Inside, everything is still. The house creaks a bit as it warms, and the table groans with the weight of my arms as I write. Wrapped in a flannel robe, my feet in thick socks, I am still cold and decide to make tea to ward off a chill.

In the middle room, in what used to be the dining room, herbs hang from the past fall's harvest, and I break off sprigs of nettles. The room is a clutter of leftover tasks lost in the rush of the holidays. A tray of rose hips waits to be stored. Bayberries, saved for candle making, wait for me to have time to use them. Hawthorn berries are finally dry enough. And the burdock root, gathered just as the ground was freezing, is dark and hard. Around the room, drying racks are empty and screens for the dehydrator stand back-to-back. The huge shallow basket that was filled with calendula is empty too, ready to be hung on the wall. In the herb closet, lots of new tinctures gleam in shiny bottles. And jars of all sizes are crammed full of the summer's harvest. On the table lies a clutter of notes to be organized. The whole room is a memory, full of stories and scents that made up the past few months, all waiting to be tucked away for a season of rest. From the herb cabinet, I take a huge jar of dried red clover blossoms. They smell sweet as spring, and I grab a few to go along with the nettles.

Back at the kitchen table now, waiting for the tea to cool, I think about the beginnings of my life on the land, back to a most precious time full of magic and miracles, and of the chain of decisions that led me here, to this house, to this window, to these fields and forests, and to herbs.

When I was a child in Louisiana, the earth seemed filled with mystery. Something in it tugged at me, something nameless, and I would stare off into any green distance with a longing that touched my heart and soul. Any wild place was a haven. At home, in the early mornings before anyone was up, I'd steal out of the house and race down to the bayou nearby. Slipping through damp fields, I would make my way to the water's edge and sit until the sun came up, watching the heavy mists rise and disappear.

At my grandmother's home on 80 acres of fields and woods bordering the Mississippi River, pecan and live oak trees shaded the yards and banana trees grew outside the kitchen door. With my father, I walked the land, listening to stories about his childhood, and learning the names of wild plants that stubbled the fields. By myself, I would wander and dream, taking a book into a low-branched tree to read, or burying myself with needles from the long leaf pines that grew alongside the old house. These times were my comfort and solace in a world that was confusing and contradictory, where rules for living seemed disconnected from what was real, and where pain was something to adapt to and ignore. In a world that seemed to make no sense, the earth took care of me, and I reveled in it.

Growing up, I learned to adjust. I put aside questions, tucked away my deeper longings, and went about the business of growing up. A marriage, a divorce, and two children later, I began a process of healing that led me back to a dream—to live on the land, to live simply and gently, and to let the earth's neutral giving help me to unfold.

With two children, all our belongings, and a car full of cats, I moved to my first country home. Neighbors were a half-mile away. Fields surrounding our house led to woods that led to our own private lake. The land had been unused for some time, and fox and skunk and deer passed close to the house often. The fields bloomed and filled with color, and the woods were filled with mysteries waiting to be discovered. Within days, our city edges wore away. Daughters, ages 10 and 12, arrived rough but were softened, and soon played together again like children.

For me, the time was a gift and a miracle. Home alone, with the kids in school, I began to explore. Up on the hill behind our place, an abandoned henhouse held field-hardy birds whose eggs I carefully carried home in a pocket. Early in the mornings, great blue herons came to the lake, and if I crept there quietly I could watch them bathe. I made friends with an otter who touched me one day nose-to-nose while I sat stone-still at the water's edge. And then he played for me, turning over and over in the water while I watched.

I worked in the soil, planting tiny seeds, becoming one simple task after another. In the joyful, mindless toil of tending the land, I relearned that life makes sense. I worked and was rewarded; I gave and reaped multitudes in return. The crazy demands of the world slid away, and the earth's magic caught me up and took me home. In the space the earth allowed me, questions became answers. I shed layers and bloomed, living in a clear, uncluttered passion. I became again a child, at one with all things. There were no secrets kept from me.

Nothing was complex or confusing. Earth and I spoke a common language, that of joy.

I explored the world around me with new eyes, and marveled at the earth's abundance. Everything we needed was already given. We simply had to look. Plants that grew just beneath our feet could be used as wild foods, or even medicine, and I set off to sample what I could find. I took home sassafras roots to simmer in water with maple syrup and drink as a spring tonic. Around an abandoned farmhouse, cleavers spread like a clingy blanket. Lady's slipper grew down a logging road, and we rescued some that would be bulldozed for a building site.

The children liked helping to gather their own medicine. It made healing tangible and familiar. I fixed poultices for their small wounds. Mullein, comfrey, and coltsfoot were used for a daughter's asthma. Weaving these easy gifts into the fabric of our everyday lives was our celebration of the earth around us. With its support, we grew healthy and flourished.

So much had been given to us in our time on the land, I longed to connect others to the earth as I had been. I began to study medicinal plants and learned to use herbs for physical problems. And I offered herb walks, still one of my favorite things to do. Now I am offering this book. It is written in journal form to chronicle each season and its herbs as they appear, spring through fall.

I keep close contact with the land around me. Each year I see something I haven't used before. Last year I found a tall meadow rue, useful in treating shingles and eczema, and a lobelia I hadn't seen before. My winter's reading has revealed that *Liatris,* the new scourge of the local countryside, has medicinal properties and that the nasturtium I use as a companion plant with my beans can also be used for colds and bronchitis. I haven't seen prickly ash yet, or stoneroot, and I'm still not sure which wild cherry I should be gathering.

But I do have an undying passion for this land. I have seen and prepared and used herbs that grow wherever I am. I offer this journal as a simple guide to using medicinal plants. And more importantly, to getting acquainted with the natural gifts around you. As human beings we make daily choices that determine the future of the environment. My hope is that as we become aware of the gifts of the earth, we will become more responsible caretakers. Perhaps this book can be one step in that awareness. And an invitation to the joy that links us all!

INTRODUCTION:
THE EARTH AS HEALER

Reflections: I met a neighbor who told me that when he was a little boy, some 60 years ago, he lived in the house where I live now. It was a boardinghouse then, and one of the boarders was a woman, about 65 or 70 years old, who knew all the plants and trees and mushrooms, all the natural things the earth has to offer. I like knowing that. It's fun to think that so long ago, some woman lived in my house who did what I do now—walk and study and watch things change and grow. I wonder what she'd think of things. I'd like to walk with her and compare notes. It's a good house, good land, and a good place to feel the earth's magic at work.

The earth's magic is profound and unfathomable, yet simple and everyday. Like a baby's smile, it touches our very hearts, reminding us of the gifts that are our birthright. In gentle neutrality, the earth affirms our worth as one tiny, but whole and beloved part of creation. The earth's abundance provides all things, often before the need is known. Her constancy renews our faith. Her balance restores a sense of harmony. And sweet joy in the earth's beauty lights our lives. In the earth's embrace, we are nourished and housed and clothed, renewed and healed.

Some gifts of the earth touch our spirits, reaching through a clutter of beliefs to return us to who we are that is good and whole. When our lives become abstract and entangled, the earth returns us to ultimate sanity. We spend time working in a garden, and cares and frustrations melt away. We cannot say exactly what it is that happens, but we are wholer. Family farmers put up with intolerable, impossible hours and odds just to live on the land. They are unable to explain what it is they get in return. Cranky, unruly children are sent outdoors to play. They come back settled and peaceful after a few hours in the fresh air and sunshine. Some of the earth's gifts are so quiet, we can easily fail to notice them. Wherever land is damaged or threatened, the earth quickly attempts repair. After fires, blueberry bushes and new birch and pine trees crowd the damaged soil, making a claim in the name of renewal. Along highways, where gases from car exhaust contaminate the air, plants absorb harmful pollutants. In slow waterways, plants act as filters, cleaning dangerous substances from the water. In our homes, plants take waste products from the air and neutralize them, giving oxygen in return. At every step, the earth works to ensure the balance necessary for survival.

Some of the earth's gifts are solid and obvious. Since time began, humans have depended upon plants to support and sustain physical life. Trees that sprout from nothing more than rock and moisture and a handful of soil become homes and provide warmth against a chill. Plants and trees offer shade and hold the soil in place. They become tools of work and implements of comfort. Trees become pulp that becomes paper that becomes a thread of communication in our abstract lives. And when plants are no longer active, they decay, enriching the soil for future generations of life and growth.

Plants serve as nourishment. Always, humankind has looked to the earth and its plants for sustenance. Most of the human population, as well as a host of other species, depend on grains and other plants as their primary food source. In early times, wild plants served as supplements, filling out diets of meat that would otherwise be incomplete. Now, cultivated vegetables and fruits, nuts and seeds supplement grains. Other foods, such as dairy and meat products, come from animals who use grains as their primary diet.

Plants are also used for healing. In simplest times, lives were intimately connected to the land. Lessons could be learned from Earth by simply observing her changes. Seasons were told on a certain wind. The color of the sky or the shape of clouds predicted rain or drought. Subtle shifts of leaves, faint scents, the ripening of pollen, the thickening of fur on beasts taken for food—all foretold changes that would impact lives. Senses were sharp and relied upon for guidance. Instinct was active and demanding, a powerful force in decision making. Animals who were weak or ill stopped eating some plants and included others. Perhaps early cultures imitated them and learned of healing plants by trial and error. Or perhaps instinct stretched so far as to lead the quiet listener to what was needed for the balance of the body.

As consciousness evolved, some cultures began to understand the earth and humankind as holy partners in life's journey. Early Native Americans saw the land and its gifts as one sacred part of a great whole whose participants were related and of equal importance. In a conscious connection with the earth, each person was his or her own healer. Plants were seen as sacred and treated with respect. And just as each member had an important individual function in the tribe, so did each plant impart some special aspect of healing.

In time, the task of healing was left to one or more individuals in the group or community. The healers maintained a close connection with the world of subtle changes. Disease was seen as an imbalance in the gentle forces of spirit that expressed themselves in physical form. To alter the disease, the gifts of the earth were employed to help move the body and spirit back toward harmony.

With the development of Western medicine, systems of healing became more sophisticated. What began as hints taken from the earth's gentle movement and flow became word of mouth. Word of mouth became documentation, which in turn became dogma. Personal curiosity and experimentation were replaced by a formal science that struggled for reason and proof. Healing became more limited to the few rather than a daily part of every person's natural life.

Soon, technology and science came to supplant traditional methods of healing. The body was seen as an intricate machine whose functions could be chemically altered or repaired. For a while, plants continued to provide chemicals necessary for healing. Then, with the development of laboratory techniques, active properties were isolated from traditionally used plants and given in place of the whole herb. As science learned to synthesize some of the plant properties, chemical drugs took the place of plant medicines.

The advantage of synthetic drugs was tremendous. The physician— the healer of modern times—could be certain of exactly how much of any one chemical was being given. And because the active properties were isolated and given in pure (or purely synthesized) form, they were more potent and predictable than the raw plant medicines of earlier times. With the refinement of pharmacological drugs, healing passed out of the hands of the individual and into the hands of trained physicians. The newly isolated and synthesized compounds were too powerful and potentially toxic for the untrained to employ. As drugs became more central to medical care, physicians and pharmaceutical firms became the new partners in healing, and reliance on plant drugs dwindled. Families came to depend on physicians who offered prescribed drugs for health, and the old traditions were forgotten.

As modern medicine became more complex, the task of physicians was so specialized that whole health care became infrequent. The doctor who had attended to the health of entire families and knew each person individually disappeared. And personal health care was so far removed from everyday life that the patient was no longer a partner in his or her own wellness. The physician assumed or was given the impossible burden of carrying all the responsibility for individual and collective health.

At the same time, in the world outside of medicine, technology inadvertently brought about specialization of other phases of daily living. The head of the family no longer worked on the farm or in the home. Labor was performed in a neutral setting, disconnected from family life. Schooling became public, and children were gone from home for long hours during the day. Populations increased, swelling small towns into cities, and the family next door was no longer related or even familiar. The fragmentation of medical care was mirrored by social anonymity and a fractured sense of community. In the name of progress, connectedness suffered. And while modern technological medicine saved countless lives that would have been lost only a short time ago, something vital was missing.

Of late, we have begun to search again for balance. We seek out or create community. Some move away from cities in favor of small towns where ties are obvious and faces are familiar. In our health care, we demand more clarity and more control. And we insist on our inherent right to heal ourselves—to take back some of the responsibility for our own wellness and to be active partners in healing. In a global world where so much distance stands between us and the vital supports of our lives, where nothing is valued unless it can be proven to have monetary value, and where often we feel like a statistic, there is a deep longing for something that makes sense to us. We long for something we can know intimately and with which we can be involved in our everyday lives. While medicinal plants are not necessarily a panacea of health care, there is something about them that sparks a hope that is difficult to define. Perhaps we are just longing for something simple and manageable in a world that seems so complex. In any case, medicinal plants have offered themselves as partners in healing since before recorded history. Even in this complex age, returning to the use of medicinal plants offers a step in the direction of reunion with the living, breathing life-form that supports us.

Of course, we do not live in simple times. Although medicinal plants still offer the same components and healing bounty they always have, as members of a Western culture we are no longer "free" to evaluate herbs in their simple reality. We approach healing not neutrally, but both blessed and burdened with a paradigm and worldview that does not allow us to evaluate simply by instinct, or by listening to and acting on what might seem reasonable to us personally. We have become dependent upon a science that can only understand what it evaluates through one particular way of seeing, and now we must wait and watch while science tries to determine how to "see" herbs.

The issue of harvesting medicinal plants, although it seems like a natural pursuit, has become complex as well. On one hand, harvesting our own plants in the wild offers a precious and simple way to participate in our surroundings and to make a tangible cycle of connection with the land in a way that both heals and nourishes our physical and spiritual lives. On the other hand, we live in times when our burden on the earth is beyond imagining. Even if we live in a rural area, chances are that the ecosystems that underlie our human lives are burdened and fragmented by the pressures of human expansion. Ecosystems are hard pressed to maintain integrity. Plant species are at risk in greater numbers than ever before, and not only in the rain forests but right beneath our feet. Humans no longer live intimately wedded to their land, and it becomes easier to not notice when the land is changed by our encroachment. So while practicing herbalism, becoming familiar with and harvesting the plants native to our regions, offers a means to get reconnected, it can also become just another threat to our "home ground."

Using proper harvesting guidelines and staying in touch with your local environmental organizations to keep abreast of plant populations and their risk status can help. Most states publish a list of endangered and threatened plants, and it is good practice to request a copy of your state's guidelines. Become familiar with those particular plants, and make certain not to harvest them. You can also make certain to utilize those local medicinal herbs that are "weedy," whose growth habits are suited to harvesting because they are present in vast numbers or seed readily. Growing medicinal plants is an option also. Find a plant you are interested in and that you know is at risk in your area, and make a space in your garden where you can encourage it. This gives you an opportunity to get to know the herb, experience its habits and needs, and eventually reintroduce it into an area where it once thrived—all part of the cycle of giving back to the earth that supports you.

When you are ready to integrate medicinal plants into your health care, they are fairly simple to introduce into everyday life. They are easy to identify and gather, and most are safe to use in moderation. Many herbs can be taken as simple teas, and some are quite tasty. Even children can help gather plants they will later use as medicine, making them partners in their own healing process.

Medicinal plants can help provide relief for minor illnesses, can help ward off more serious complications, and show promise in preventive medicine as well. They also work in subtle ways to help balance body systems. They can be useful in correcting annoying conditions that are not full-blown disease and for which we would not normally seek out medical care. They also generally produce far fewer side effects than synthetic drugs, an important consideration in the search for balance.

Of course, there are no instant cures for any physical problem. Nutrition, exercise, and attitude are all important factors, with each contributing its own sense of sanity and balance to our wellness process. And it is crucial to be mindful of your limits. Some health problems are well within your ability to cope, and for others you will need professional help. Herbs offer some vital beginning and intermediate steps in health care, and conventional medicine provides relief from life-threatening or disabling conditions. Each process has an essential place in the pursuit of wellness, and each reflects an important aspect of our needs and skills as human beings. The conscious integration of each form of healing is an important part of achieving balance.

In whatever way you decide to participate in the world of medicinal plants, healing is available for each of us. Earth and her precious gifts are always there, ready to touch a secret place in us that opens doors. Earth's magic is our magic too, forgotten or tucked away. The earth simply acts as a reminder. And the magic is what keeps us going. It sparks our very being and takes us home again.

The following pages present information to help you begin exploring the earth's bounty. A cycle of steps is described, from identification of plants and details of harvesting, through making simple preparations, and then using the herbs. Journal notes in each section will lead you through one person's experiences and offer some of nature's clues to what each season might reveal as you search for plants.

While all the herbs in this book were found and harvested in the New England area, they are certainly not limited to the Northeast. Many are common throughout the United States and have been used by Native healers in local regions for ages. The herbs described are not a comprehensive listing, but a sampling of plants, chosen for their relative safety and simplicity of use. Various species of the plants mentioned can be found in the South, in the Midwest and the Pacific Northwest, in the Plains states, and even in the moister areas of semi-arid western states.

Familiarize yourself with the herbs that grow around you, and begin to integrate them into your everyday health care. Hopefully, wherever you live, this book can serve to guide you to your own deep and fruitful connection with the magical place we call home.

USING HERBS IN
THE HEALING PROCESS

Reflections: How much I change things when I harvest plants! Even gathering something as abundant as chickweed or violets, I change worlds. Next year, chickweed may not grow where I pulled it up; the violet will not have the same neighbor. The responsibility is awesome, but somewhere along the line, I seem to have gotten permission from Earth to use her gifts. I will gather with gratitude and awareness and caution as to supply. I'm part of the natural life, too, and hopefully I will be gentle in my willfulness and keep whatever harmony I can.

GATHERING YOUR PLANTS

At first, harvesting herbs may seem hard to do. It's one thing to bring home a single plant to look up in the herbals and plant guides and learn about it, and another to harvest plants for use. Harvesting means batches. It sometimes means killing a plant, and not just one, but many. Some simple rules, though, will ensure that you, the land, and the plants you gather remain healthy and vigorous.

First, harvest only plants with which you are familiar or that you can identify with certainty. Look through the identification sections of this book or through your local plant guides, and compare their notes with the features of the plant you intend to harvest. There will be variations from plant to plant, but generally the major points described should match your specimen. If you are unsure of the name of a plant, gather a few sprigs and save them in a plant press, along with the date and location. You may later run into information that enables you to identify the specimen, and you will want to know where to find the plant again should you want to gather it.

Second, if you are gathering on your own land, make an informal survey of the plant life over a period of time. You will want to be sure that the plant you are gathering isn't just an isolated specimen. If the plants in the population are healthy looking, recur every year, and grow in more than one place, it is safe to assume that the plant is not in danger of being eradicated if you harvest some. It is also best to know which plants are scarce in your region. You can obtain a list of your state's rare or endangered plants from your natural resource agency or from your local Audubon Society to help you make decisions about what to gather.

If you are harvesting on land other than your own, make reasonably sure there are no nearby sources of pollution, and if you gather plants along a roadside, be certain that the road is not heavily traveled. Plants exposed to heavy traffic absorb pollutants expelled by automobiles and should not be used. Also, determine whether the area has been sprayed for weed control. Obtain landowner's permission if possible, too. Many landowners are more than glad to have someone get rid of the "weeds," but it is best to check beforehand to avoid hard feelings or even arrest for trespassing.

Wherever you harvest your herbs, gather only healthy-looking plants, and pick out any discolored or insect-damaged plant parts before making your preparations.

Harvest Timing

The best times for harvesting plant parts vary, but some general guidelines can be applied.

Whole plants—such as shepherd's purse—or plants whose aboveground parts will be used—such as the mints—should be harvested when plant growth is lush and the plant is just starting to blossom. Pull whole plants at the base, and for aboveground parts of plants, cut the stems a few inches above the ground, and bind them together at the base.

Leaves to be used should be gathered when the plant is in healthy and vigorous growth. For some plants, this time period extends throughout the growing season. For instance, raspberry leaves are green in early summer through the first frosts. Because the plant is in peak growth when it is first starting to flower, leaves gathered then may have higher medicinal potency, but in general the leaves will be useful any time they are healthy looking.

Blossoms of plants to be used should be picked when they are just opening. Fruits, such as hawthorn berries or rose hips, are gathered when they are ripe and colorful. Rose hips are best after a first frost.

Bark is generally gathered in the spring as the plant begins its new growth. (An exception is the wild cherry, whose medicinal content is highest in the fall.)

Roots and *root bark* can be gathered in early spring when plants have barely begun their seasonal growth spurt or in fall after the first few frosts. In autumn, leaf material dies back and plant compounds are concentrated in the roots for winter.

CAUTIONS: There are two cautions to be exercised if gathering spring roots. First, plant identification in the spring can be somewhat tricky, since very little leaf material is available. Mistakes are easy to make. A good step to take if you are planning to gather roots in spring is to mark the plant with bright twine or some other indicator the previous fall, and then gather only those roots you have marked.

Second, in spring, the sugar content in the roots tends to be higher. This increased sugar content can make roots harder to dry and more susceptible to rot if drying conditions are not optimal.

Drying Your Plants

Careful and quick drying are the keys to insuring that the plant you have gathered will be potent and useful for as long as possible. Most drying of herbs is best done in a shaded, warm, well-ventilated space where humidity is low. A second-story room or an airy attic are good sites. If neither of these is available, a hanging space close to the ceiling of a shaded room is good. In very humid weather, air drying may be difficult, and an electric food dehydrator can be used to dry herbs quickly and prevent molding.

Another option is to oven dry your herbs. In a gas range, plant parts may be spread out on a cookie sheet and simply placed in the oven with the pilot light on. If using an electric oven, set the temperature control to its lowest reading (or WARM), and prop the door ajar to allow moisture to escape. A wood-burning stove could probably be used if you can maintain a very low (just over 100 degrees) and constant temperature.

Bundle *leafy or flowering plants,* such as the mints, together and rinse under running water to remove loose dirt. Bind the stems together with a rubber band at the bases, and hang the bundles to dry, keeping them out of the sun or strong light. (Rubber bands will shrink in size along with the plant parts as they dehydrate.) The plants will dry in 1–2 weeks, depending on the humidity, air temperature, and the water content of the plants gathered. A good test for complete dryness is to take the plant between thumb and fingers and press it. If the plant parts crumble to the touch, they're ready to be stored.

Large, flat leaf clusters, such as raspberry leaves, or fleshier individual leaves, such as coltsfoot, can be spread out on screening material or cheesecloth stretched over a simple wooden frame. They may also be spread out in the flat bottom of shallow, wide-weave baskets. Brown paper bags opened and spread out will also do. The leaves should be laid one layer thick. Fleshy leaves should be turned every day or so to ensure good air exposure on both sides.

Small whole plants, such as violets or pipsissewa, can be dried like individual leaves, with each plant spread out on a screen or basket and turned every day or so. Individual blossoms such as red clover heads can also be dried using this method and should also be turned.

To prepare *roots* for drying, clean them immediately and slice as thinly as possible. Spread on screens, baskets, brown paper bags, or on cheesecloth hung along a collapsible clothes-drying rack. Root material may then be set outdoors in a sunny spot for the first day or two, where the sun will cure, or seal, the exposed cut surfaces and hasten drying. Turn the pieces of root over occasionally to ensure curing on both sides. At night, or if damp weather threatens, bring root material indoors. After a day or two, roots should be sealed and can be brought indoors to complete the drying process. As is to be expected, root material may take longer to dry than leafy plant parts. Roots that are truly dry will snap between thumb and fingers when pressure is applied. Plant *barks* can be dried in this manner also.

Dry *fruits and berries* by spreading a single layer on screens, flattened paper bags, or baskets. Set them in a shaded area, away from the sun. To test for dryness, cut open a few and inspect them well to make sure no moisture remains. Fleshier fruits such as rose hips may be difficult to dry if conditions are not optimal. In this case, an electric food dehydrator can be used, or the herbs can be oven dried. Simply spread the fruit, one layer thick, on a cookie sheet or dehydrator tray. Check every half-hour or so for dryness, which will be indicated by dark, hard brittleness of the fruit. Fleshier fruit may take hours to dry. These methods can also be used for root material.

Storing Your Herbs

Because light, heat, and air can alter the chemical components of most plants, the best storage for all herbs and herbal products is in air-tight glass or ceramic containers, in a dark, fairly cool environment, such as a cabinet. If amber glass can be obtained, it should be used, for it filters out light. Otherwise, glass canning jars are fine, if you keep them out of the sun.

Dried herbs will remain stable for varying lengths of time. Six months to one year is a general time frame for viability, although if well dried and stored, some herbs may last longer. Other herbs may be unstable in a dried state, and it is useful to tincture herbs that you will not be using for a long time.

All stored herbs should be labeled with their common and Latin names, as well as the dates they were gathered and processed. When you are ready to use the herb, taste and sniff it for freshness and flavor, and examine it for color. If it seems dull and tasteless, it is probably not worth using. Replenish your supply of dried herbs every year.

Making Your Preparations

Part of the fun of using herbs is making preparations with what you have gathered and stored. As you begin to experiment, you become more familiar with the herb. There is time to see how it withstands the passage of time, how it reconstitutes with liquid, and how it tastes as it changes into a tea or tincture or syrup.

Equipment

You can make most of the herbal preparations listed in this book with simple kitchen tools or things you might normally have around the house. Items that you will need include:

- a pair of scissors or shears
- a sharp knife
- a blender or mortar and pestle,
- a glass measuring vessel with milliliters marked on the side
- a simple postal scale
- a stainless steel or glass cooking pot
- coffee filters
- cheesecloth
- glass or ceramic jars with tight-fitting lids
- labels or tags
- a tea ball or bamboo tea strainer

Supplies include:

- beeswax
- grain alcohol, high-proof vodka or cider vinegar, or glycerin
- high-quality oil such as olive or almond
- honey
- rubbing alcohol
- cayenne pepper

Teas

Herbal teas may be made from fresh or dried plant materials—leaves, blossoms, roots, bark, or fruit, or a combination of these.

A new cup of tea may be made for each dose taken or a large amount may be made ahead of time and drunk throughout the day. Any tea made ahead, though, should be refrigerated, and then just the right amount reheated when you are ready to use it. Most teas should be drunk while they are hot or warm, but specific variations are listed in each plant's dosage section later in this book.

There are two basic ways of making a tea. In an *infusion,* the plant compounds are extracted by pouring boiling water directly over the plant material, which is immersed in the hot water with a bamboo strainer, stainless steel ball or spoon, or reusable cloth tea bag. A general rule of thumb for making infusions is to use 1 tablespoon of dried herb to 1 cup of boiling water, and steep for 15–30 minutes. Since variations do exist for each plant, check the specific directions for individual herbs. If using fresh herbs, double the amount of plant material, as its water content will be much higher and so the tea less concentrated.

When plant matter is woody, as with roots and bark, a *decoction* is made. In this form of tea, the plant materials are placed directly into the water before heating. The water is then brought to a boil, and the mixture is simmered for a few minutes. The plant material is strained out before the tea is drunk. If making a tea with a blend of both roots and leafy herbs, make the decoction first, simmering the plant parts for the suggested time. Then, remove from heat and place leafy herbs into the hot decoction for several minutes. Strain out all plant parts, and drink the tea as suggested.

Tinctures

A *tincture* is a concentrated herbal preparation in which a liquid other than water has been used to extract medicinal components from the fresh or dried plant. Following preparation, the herb is discarded, and the resulting tincture is stored for later use.

Tinctures have a few advantages over teas. One of these is stability. Once a plant has been tinctured, the extraction liquid acts to preserve the plant components, thereby making it useful indefinitely. Another asset of tinctures is that the medium used for extraction can break down oily or resinous compounds in some plants that would not be so available with hot water.

The three most commonly used mediums of extraction are high-proof drinking alcohol (as opposed to rubbing alcohol), natural glycerin, and cider vinegar. Each has advantages and disadvantages, but all, to varying degrees, will serve to extract and preserve medicinal properties of plant materials. There are different schools of thought about which liquid is most appropriate. Since all will produce a useful product, the choice remains a personal one, based on your needs, values, and lifestyle.

Alcohol is very effective at breaking down and preserving plant compounds that won't dissolve simply in water. These compounds are often oily or resinous and do not become available even with applied heat, such as with boiling or steeping in hot water. Because alcohol is so effective at breaking down heavier plant properties, the resulting tincture is very concentrated and only small doses of it are taken at a time. In addition to alcohol's effectiveness in dissolving plant properties, it acts as a preservative, leaving the plant medicine stable for years. Alcohol is also absorbed into the bloodstream readily, making the medicinal properties available to the body shortly after ingestion.

The disadvantages of alcohol are fairly obvious. The use of alcohol in excess, or even in small doses for some people, can produce unwanted effects. Also, when using herbs for children, palatability is often a major factor. Since alcohol is an acquired taste, it is likely to be rejected more often than not by children unless the taste is disguised.

Glycerin is a chemical compound based on combined molecules of sugar, fatty acid, and alcohol. It has a much lower potential for extraction of medicinal components than does alcohol, but is especially effective at extracting such fat-based substances as natural hormones in plants. Glycerin has an added advantage of being sweet tasting, making it more acceptable to children. Because the potency of glycerin is lower than that of alcohol, dosage of glycerin tinctures is usually increased three to four times the normal dose of an alcohol based tincture (for example, instead of 30 drops, which is about $1/4$ teaspoon of tincture, you might take a 100–120 drops, or a whole teaspoon of tincture, at a time.).

Cider vinegar is a fermented form of the cider pressed from apples. It acts to extract some of the oily or resinous properties of plants by virtue of its acidity, which ranges from 5 percent to 14 percent. It will also act to preserve the plant preparation. Cider vinegar is metabolized easily in the body and has been traditionally used as a tonic thought to stimulate digestion and to have healing properties of its own.

An advantage of using vinegar to make tinctures is that there is virtually no toxicity associated with cider vinegar taken in moderate quantity. Another advantage to vinegar is that it is thought of as a food product, and its use can be integrated into everyday life. The chief disadvantage of using cider vinegar as an extraction medium is its low potency. The highest available acidity in cider vinegar is 14 percent, which means that the liquid is 86 percent water. Thus, vinegar has a very low potential for extraction compared to alcohol.

Plants may be tinctured either fresh or dried. Generally, I prefer to make fresh-plant tinctures, since this means that the resulting preparation will have as much of the medicinal compounds of the plant as the tincture medium can extract. With drying, generally some potency is lost in the drying process, and the resulting tincture may not be as effective as if the plant were processed as soon as it was harvested. However, dried plant tinctures are also effective, and I often end up making both during the course of a year.

Fresh-plant tinctures: In making a fresh-plant tincture, the proportions are measured by volume, and are basically one part plant to one part liquid. In this method, the plant is harvested and cleaned, removing any damaged leaves or blossoms and washing very carefully if the root is used. Chop or cut the plant material into very small pieces, and place in a glass jar. Pour the liquid to be used for extraction directly over the plant material in the jar until it just barely covers the herb. If desired, you can place a smooth, clean stone on top of the plant to keep it beneath the level of the liquid. Tightly cap the jar, and place it in a cabinet or other cool, dark place for two to six weeks, shaking every day or so to allow good exposure of all plant parts to liquid. (While alcohol can extract the compounds effectively within two weeks, both glycerin and vinegar require about six weeks.) After the plant has set for an appropriate time, pour off and strain the liquid—now your tincture—through several layers of cheesecloth or through coffee filters. The leftover plant material can be placed in damp cheesecloth and squeezed tightly to obtain any remaining tincture. The spent plant material can be discarded or added to your compost, and your tincture should be bottled, labeled, and stored.

A double extraction can also be made with fresh-plant tinctures, especially if you are using glycerin or cider vinegar as a medium. After the first tincture has set for two to six weeks, simply gather another batch of the fresh herb, prepare it by chopping into small bits, and place it into a jar. Then, instead of covering it with fresh glycerin or cider vinegar, pour the original tincture over it, cover the jar, and store for two more weeks.

Dried-Plant Tinctures: Traditionally, a 50/50 mixture of alcohol and water has proved most effective at extracting water-soluble and non-water-soluble properties of most dried plants. Vodka can be purchased at 110 proof, which is 55 percent alcohol. Since most plants will release their properties in a mixture of 50 percent alcohol and 50 percent water, this percentage in vodka is ideal for making tinctures from dried plant materials. The alcohol content will work to extract oily properties, and the water will rehydrate the plant and extract water-soluble properties. To make your dried-plant, alcohol-based tincture, chop the plant material in a blender or crush by hand using a mortar and pestle until you have a coarse powder. Weigh the powder using a home postal scale, and record the weight in grams. To the crushed herb, add five times its weight in liquid. For example, if you have 50 grams of powdered herb, you will want to add 250 milliliters of high-proof vodka. (Milliliters, abbreviated ml, are marked clearly on the sides of some glass measuring cups; a milliliter of liquid measure is equal to a gram, or g, in dry measure.) When you have measured out the proper amount of liquid, place the crushed herb in a jar and pour the alcohol over it. Close the jar and shake the mixture vigorously. Then set the jar in a cool, dark place, such as a cabinet, for two weeks. During that time, shake the jar occasionally to allow for good exposure of plant to liquid.

After two weeks, remove the lid and pour the mixture through a fine sieve or through layers of cheesecloth. The liquid should then be strained through a coffee filter to remove all plant debris. The spent herb can be placed in damp cheesecloth and squeezed hard to extract as much of the remaining tincture as possible. The herb is then discarded, and the tincture bottled in a ceramic or glass vessel, tightly capped, labeled, and stored.

To make a tincture using cider vinegar as the extraction liquid, the procedure is the same as that described for alcohol. Weigh the crushed herb and place it in a jar, along with five times its weight in cider vinegar. Seal and shake the jar, and tuck it away for two to six weeks. Strain and filter as described above. To increase the potency of the tincture, you may wish to do a double extraction. To do this, pour off your original tincture and prepare a new batch of dried herb. This time, follow the same procedure, but use the tincture you have just produced for your extraction liquid, thereby doubling the content of plant properties in the final tincture. If you choose to follow this procedure, be sure to measure the liquid and the dried herb carefully before starting the second tincture. You will probably have less liquid than you started with originally, as some of it will have been reabsorbed by the dried plant in its rehydration.

If making a glycerin tincture from dried plant material, you will have to add some water to the dried herb to rehydrate it. Generally, this should be 20 percent of the liquid. For instance, if using 100 ml of liquid, use 20 ml of water and 80 ml of glycerin. Mix water and glycerin together and pour over the herb. Proceed as in alcohol and cider vinegar tincture making, shaking vigorously and then setting aside for two to six weeks.

Syrups

A *syrup* is a way of preparing herbs so that they taste good and are soothing to the membranes of the throat. My favorite syrup base is local honey, which comes from bees who work the local flowers and herbs. Honey is soothing and healing in itself and is also nutritious. Local honey has the further advantage of helping to provide immunities to regional plant pollens. As a sweetener, honey also serves to preserve the herbs used in it. Shelf life of honey-based syrups varies, but they should be dependable for several years.

To make a syrup using honey, simply place dried plant material in a pot, and cover with honey. The proportions are generally one part plant matter to one part honey. Simmer the mixture on very low heat on the stove, without a lid, for half an hour, stirring often to keep the mixture from boiling.

Another method of making syrup is to use a Crock-Pot with the heat setting adjusted to just above 100 degrees. Place all plant matter into the Crock-Pot and cover with honey. Allow this mixture to stew uncovered for 5–24 hours at the same very low temperature. Following preparation of your syrup, remove the plant material and strain the liquid through several layers of clean cheesecloth. Pour the hot syrup into sterile jars, and label with contents and date. The jars should then be placed into a dark, cool cabinet for storage.

Salves

A *salve* is a method of using herbs that enables you to keep the plant in close, constant contact with the skin. Generally, cold-pressed olive oil is the best medium for herbal salves, although other high-quality oils will do fine. Beeswax is used to solidify the salve as it is a natural product and has healing properties of its own. The simplest salve involves placing dried plant material, such as comfrey leaves, into a jar. Pour in a good-quality oil, such as cold-pressed olive or almond oil, until the plant parts are just covered. To this mixture, add a natural preservative to keep the oil from getting rancid. For this, you may use either the contents of a couple of vitamin E oil capsules, or $1/2$ teaspoon of tincture of benzoin, available from a local pharmacy. (Benzoin has a strong medicinal smell that will affect the scent of the finished product.) Stir the mixture well, cap the jar, and place it in a warm spot for two weeks. At the end of this time period, strain the mixture first through a sieve and then through cheesecloth, and discard any plant matter. Measure the remaining herbal oil in a glass measuring cup and record the amount in milliliters. To this herbal oil, add $1/4$ the amount of oil in beeswax. For example, if you have 200 milliliters of herbal oil, add 50 grams of beeswax to the oil. Heat the oil and beeswax in the pot on low setting until the beeswax is thoroughly melted, stirring occasionally to ensure proper mixing. Use caution, as all waxes are flammable. Remove from heat and pour into containers. Allow to cool thoroughly before covering with lids.

The proportions of oil to beeswax are flexible and may vary according to your personal preference. More beeswax will produce a more solid salve, and less will result in a softer product.

Liniment

A *liniment* is an herbal product in liquid form that is applied externally for the purpose of being absorbed into deeper tissues. It is often used along with gentle massage to injured or bruised areas where there is no broken skin. The base of a liniment is generally rubbing alcohol, witch hazel, or cider vinegar. These will all act to break down plant components and to preserve them.

To make a liniment, chop plant material, such as wintergreen leaves, into small pieces—about $1/2$ inch long—and place in an empty 1 quart jar. If desired, add $1/2$ teaspoon of cayenne pepper. (The pepper acts as a stimulant, increasing circulation to the area, and aids the skin in absorbing the plant properties.) Pack the herb down, using a stone on top to keep the plant immersed in alcohol if necessary. Pour in enough liquid to cover the herb, and close the jar. Shake gently to allow good exposure of the herb to the alcohol. Place the jar in a cabinet out of the sun, and shake every few days. After two weeks, shake well and strain off the liquid, now your liniment. Discard the herb. To use liniment, apply directly to skin for muscle and joint soreness or bruises, strains, and strains. The liniment may be applied to a clean cloth and kept in place over the affected area for 10–15 minutes several times a day if needed.

These suggestions provide enough basic information for you to use the herbs in this book in various ways. But do not feel limited by them. The nature of herbalism is experimentation. Within the firm margins of safety, let yourself be guided by the plants and by your own instinct. Remember that herbs are potent medicine and their use requires that you be respectful of your body and of the plants. Above all, know that your wellness is one of your natural birthrights and that healing comes from within. The plants are simply helpers, ready to guide you toward your own internal balance.

SPRING

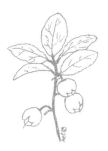

WILLOW
Salix species

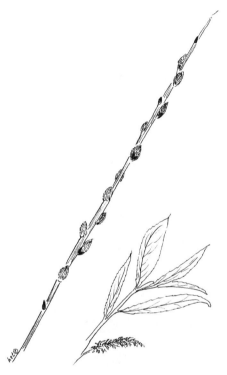

Reflections: I move from one willow tree to another and strip the bark. The sun has come up over the ridge of trees, and the woods smell wonderful—sun on pine needles. Not much moves. A red squirrel chatters at me, and somewhere close by a ruffed grouse drums his mating call. I suddenly realize that I am no longer worried about hurting the trees. Holding the bough under my chin, all I am is this work—bending and stripping, bending and stripping. I feel like a cellist playing a delightful, deep instrument that is somehow part of my body.

Description: A number of willow species occur in New England, and all can be used for the same purposes. *Salix nigra* is the traditional species for herbal use, but in general, all the willows have similar compounds.

Willows may be found as shrubs or small trees, rarely exceeding 80 feet in height. The plant may have a single, central trunk that branches off, or most often, it will have several trunks that sprout from the base. The willows are found mostly in moist areas and are common along waterways. Most of the willows have a distinct odor that can be noted upon crushing the leaves or bark.

Willow leaves, in general, are long and lance shaped with a pointed tip, and they are slightly toothed. Most flowers of the willow species occur along catkins that erupt from a scale along the branch. Seeds of the various species are generally attached to silky hairs that aid in dispersing them on the wind.

The bark of the willows ranges from gray to brown and is aromatic and bitter tasting. In small plants, the bark is smooth, but may become rough and furrowed in older or larger species. Refer to plant guides for more detailed descriptions of the various species.

Medicinal Uses: The willows contain salicin, a compound used as the base in the production of aspirin. Therefore, willow bark and twigs can be used in situations that might normally call for that drug.

Specifically, willow is anti-inflammatory and can help relieve pain and inflammation. These properties make it useful in treating headaches or arthritic pain. It can be used to help reduce pain in bladder inflammations or infections. Because of its anti-inflammatory properties, willow can be used to help reduce fevers during colds or influenza. It is also helpful in some allergic reactions, such as hay fever, where it acts to reduce swelling and inflammation of membranes.

Willow is also antiseptic, and a poultice of the freshly crushed bark or twigs can be used externally for mild scratches or wounds.

Varieties of poplar may be used in place of willow, as they are in the same plant family and share the same compounds.

Harvesting: Strip the bark from the tree or shrub in early spring as the new growth starts, or break off small twigs from the ends of branches. Spread the bark out to dry on screens or other appropriate material. Bundle the twigs and hang to dry. When the plant material breaks easily, it is ready to store.

Dosages: Use 1 tablespoon of dried, shredded willow bark or twigs. Place in 1 cup of boiling water, and simmer over low heat for 10–15 minutes. Strain out plant material, and drink three times a day.

CAUTION: People who have aspirin allergies or sensitivities should avoid using willow internally.

FROM THE AUTHOR'S JOURNAL
APRIL 5

At 5:30 AM the fat, orange half-moon is just setting. I go out to watch the Big Dipper fade as color seeps into the eastern sky. As the moon dips behind the mountain, birds begin to waken and sing—even at 5:30—and in the field behind the house, they dive and swoop for the bugs that are newly born. Across the road, frogs are beginning to chirp. The sweet high sound carries up to the hill, and the air is full of song and sleepy winds and the smell of snow melting.

Yesterday, we worked in the yard, clearing up last year's debris and turning over the garden beds. I know it's early yet and I should wait, but everything seems so eager I have to do at least a little. Like the daylily shoots standing bright green against the yellowy browns and grays of winter-tired grasses, everything is celebrating the first days of spring.

Out to be part of the celebration, I trek out to gather some smooth bark of willow. In early spring, all the trees are putting out new shoots and the medicine will be highest in the bark and twigs now. Also, the cut places in the trees I work on will have time to heal before winter threatens again.

I walk down past a neighbor's farm to Big Sandy—the hill that slopes so sharply toward the lake—to where I picked sprigs of pussy willow earlier this season. In the woods, the air smells like spring, with a thin edge of cold that gives way to damp earth and dew and new green. After a while, I decide that finding a willow to work on is harder than I expected. Finally, I find what I know is an overdone willow catkin and examine the whole sapling, pulling its branches apart from its neighbors and looking at every part. The green leaf shoots are folded against the bark in the same way the first fluff of catkins were earlier, and at the base of every sprig of leaves is a small brown scale from which the catkin emerged. In some places the first leaves are beginning to open.

I try my first sapling. The drawknife skims along the side of the greenish branch, and a thin strip of bark peels back. It is gray on the outside, and pale whitish green on the inside. It pulls off easily. I try peeling more, and then, sure I am gathering the right thing, I find a young tree whose branches are as thick as my thumb. I bend it toward me, hold it under my chin, and begin way down at the base, skimming toward me along one side. This is the first time I've taken bark from a live tree, and I can't help feeling that this must hurt the tree somehow. But I only strip the bark from one side of each sapling. This way, even though the living tissue is interrupted, at least I know I am not killing the tree. It will have time to repair the damage I've inflicted before winter comes, and to protect itself from insect damage or disease.

I get into a little rhythm with the work—bend, pull, strip, into pocket—again and again. I pop a fresh green strip into my mouth. It is intensely astringent, but there's something about it I like, so I keep chewing.

I want to stay and work at this until I'm tired, 'til my pockets are full, but it's a workday. There are chores to be done, breakfast to fix, birds to feed, exercises to do, and a million more things waiting for me. So, I leave with a full pocket and a glad heart, knowing I'll come back to watch the baby leaves unfold as the summer warms things up.

Experiences with Willow

Last year I took willow for the first time. A fierce and unusual headache struck one day and made me feel sick. There was no aspirin in the house, but I had a jar full of willow bark given to me by a friend. I simmered a small handful of the strips in boiling water for a few minutes. The tea tasted bitter, but I drank it anyway, a few swallows at a time. Half an hour later, singing through household chores, I remembered my headache. The willow seemed to have worked wonders; I even think it improved my mood. Since then, it is willow I reach for when pain strikes.

Another time, the black flies discovered me in the garden in the first sun after a string of wet and cloudy days. I rubbed at a bite on my ear for a while and then decided to try something for it. Remembering that willow is anti-inflammatory and good for pain, too, I rubbed some freshly made tincture on the itchy, burning place. It stung for a moment and then stopped. Later I realized I had forgotten about the bite, and when I checked it, there was no redness or swelling, and the itching was gone. Again, willow surprised me, working so fast and so gently I forgot all about the pain.

WINTERGREEN
Gaultheria procumbens

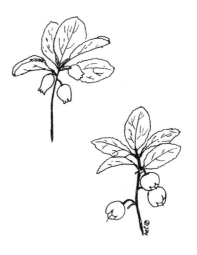

Reflections: As I leave the woods, early morning sun shines from a blue sky crowded with dark clouds. My pockets are stuffed. I have not come to gather anything today, but wintergreen seems to have offered itself. Sometimes I think it's the wonderful smell of crushed wintergreen that makes me feel so good when I am here, but I guess it really doesn't matter. I am just grateful for this protected place, for the silence and the wintergreen and the healing it offers.

Description: Wintergreen (also known as teaberry or checkerberry) is a low-growing perennial evergreen of hardwood or conifer forests. It has aromatic leaves and fruit and is often seen as the shiny green undergrowth in woodlands. It can be found under snow cover in winter.

The leaves grow in an alternate fashion but appear as a whorl atop a stiff branch rising from the creeping stem that trails at ground level. Leaves are oval or egg shaped, a bit longer than they are wide—up to 2 inches in length and 1 inch in width. They are dark green and glossy on the surface and paler and dull underneath. The margins are slightly toothed. Leaves may become burnished and can be found in a maroon or dark red color where they have been exposed to sunlight or have been hit by a sudden frost.

Wintergreen flowers are white, or pinkish white. They are bell shaped and are composed of a five-lobed corolla with a constricted tip and five small teeth that flare out from the constricted lobes. Blossoms are about $^1/_4$ to $^1/_3$ inch long and hang in loose nodding clusters from the leaf axils. They are most often found underneath the leaves, hanging in groups of one to three blossoms, although some plants bear more. Wintergreen blooms spring through early summer.

The fruit is a bright crimson berry that can be found on the plant in fall through winter and into the following spring. The edible berry has a strong wintergreen flavor, although it is somewhat mealy in texture.

Medicinal Uses: Wintergreen's primary medicinal property is methyl salicylate, which is the basic compound of aspirin. The plant is analgesic and astringent and is used internally or externally to help relieve pain.

Externally, liniment of the herb can be applied to arthritic or rheumatic joint inflammations where it may help reduce pain and irritation. The liniment is also useful for strained or sore muscles and can be applied along with gentle massage to relieve aching.

Internally, wintergreen tea can be taken for general relief of minor pains. It may be helpful in treating headaches, in the discomfort of arthritis or rheumatism, or in muscle aches and pains after strenuous exercise. Since wintergreen is also diuretic and antiseptic, it can be taken internally for mild bladder irritations where there is pain. In this case, wintergreen can help increase the flow of urine while easing the pain associated with the condition.

The oil of wintergreen, which can be purchased from an herb or health food store, can be applied to painful teeth and gums with some relief. The oil should be used sparingly, as it is very concentrated and can be toxic if swallowed.

Harvesting: Gather wintergreen when the plant is in bloom. And choose only fresh, healthy-looking leaves. Pluck leaves from each branch, or pick entire plants and bundle to dry. If gathering the leaves, spread them out on screens, paper bags, or baskets, and keep them out of the sun. Because the leaves are somewhat fleshy, wintergreen may take longer than other plants to dry. The plant is ready to store when a leaf snaps easily between fingers.

Dosages: For a tea, use 1 tablespoon of the leaves to a cup of boiling water. Cover and let steep for 15–30 minutes, then drink three times a day for pain relief or for bladder irritations. If using the oil of wintergreen for painful teeth, place a drop on the finger and apply externally to the affected tooth. The application can be repeated three or four times daily.

CAUTION: Wintergreen, especially the oil, should be avoided by those with known aspirin allergies or by people with sensitivities to many substances.

FROM THE AUTHOR'S JOURNAL
APRIL 10

I take a little walk across the road and into the woods where the forest floor is a carpet of so many shades of magic: browns layered with tans and see-through beech leaves and delicate rust-colored pine needles— all with new green balsam shoots poking through. Partridgeberry, still full of scarlet berries from last fall, laces through it all. In the tiny stream, watercress has begun to spread, and mounds of new moss are so green they seem to vibrate.

Farther back, the mosses carpet a path I walk along. My steps are padded. I imagine myself an animal, making no noise, disturbing nothing. I squat and run a hand over the moss. It is full of tiny flowers. My fingers sink into it, and I think how lovely the moss would be to sleep on. Maybe when the weather warms, I'll come back here to camp. Animals could pad quietly around me all night long.

Just beyond the moss, wintergreen covers the ground. Its shiny green leaves spread everywhere. I pluck a fresh green one and chew it up a bit, loving the flavor. Then I tuck it in my cheek, holding the leaf against a sore place on my gum. Maybe the aspirin in this plant will help. I settle into the patch, picking more leaves and filling my pockets.

Beneath me, the soft earth is marked with deer prints. Above, the tops of the pines sway in a circle, blowing in a new wind. Far away, chickadees talk. Two of them come closer and closer, circling to see what I am doing here. They are brave and curious and come within inches of me, and we chatter together for a while.

Soon, wind that started earlier blows furiously, moaning through the trees. As I get up to leave, the sore place on my gum is less tender and I am thankful that the earth knew I needed wintergreen today.

Kitchen Notes

At home, I spread the wintergreen out on the table and pick through it, throwing out bug-bitten or imperfect leaves. Some of the best leaves go into a quart jar, and I pour rubbing alcohol over them for a wintergreen liniment. The jar goes on a shelf in the herb cabinet where it will sit for a couple of weeks.

The rest of the leaves get spread out on screens to dry for tea through the seasons, for healing, or just for the wonderful flavor.

Experiences with Wintergreen

Last year I tried wintergreen in a salve for blackfly and other bug bites, and it worked fine. The pain and swelling lessened, and the itching didn't bother me as much. Friends who tried it asked for more this year.

Catnip
Nepeta cataria

Reflections: I finally finish transplanting the catnip, with its wrinkly, fuzzy leaves, to the special place I've cleared in the garden where it can spread into the field and go wild again. I wonder how soon my cat friends will find it and roll on it and smash it down, but I'm too tired to worry. I have dirt all over me. The fingernails I worked so hard at are chipped and dirty, my overalls are muddy, and my shoes are caked with soil. My daughter tells me I have dirt on my nose, but I feel too peaceful to care. The woods, the fields, the garden, and catnip all do that to me.

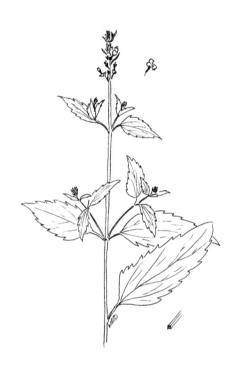

Description: Catnip is a perennial member of the Mint family. Like many of its relatives, it seeds freely and, if allowed, will take over areas where it grows. The plant is found in the wild in fields and waste places and around barns and houses. It can be easily cultivated in the garden, where care must be taken to control its growth.

Catnip has opposing leaves that are triangular shaped, coarsely toothed, and up to 3 inches long. Leaves and square stems are covered with soft downy hairs. In the wild, catnip will grow to 3 feet in height. When crushed, the plant gives off a somewhat disagreeable odor that attracts cats. The scent is not, however, typically minty.

The flowers of catnip plants are small, up to only $1/2$ inch long, and are white to pinkish white with purple spots. Blossoms occur atop the main stems and branches. Catnip flowers from early summer through the first frosts in fall.

Medicinal Uses: The dried leaves and blossoms of catnip are the parts used medicinally. Catnip has been employed traditionally for upset stomach and intestinal gas pains and especially for colic in infants. It is carminative, helping to decrease the formation of intestinal gas and to aid the body in dispelling gas that has formed. It is also antispasmodic and helps to prevent or relieve menstrual cramping.

Catnip is diaphoretic and is used to produce a natural sweat, which is helpful in lowering fevers. It is mildly sedative, too, and can be used to relieve tension and induce a restful state in infants, children, or adults.

Catnip's antispasmodic and diaphoretic properties, along with its carminative action, contribute to its usefulness in infant colic and in stomach upsets. As far as is known, the plant has no toxicity and can be used safely by infants, children, or adults, unless allergy to the plant is suspected.

Harvesting: Catnip can be gathered any time throughout its growing season, but the plant is probably highest in volatile oils just before flowering. Gather the top one-third to one-half of the stems, and bundle them together in small batches. Hang upside down to dry in an airy, shaded place. When crumbly to the touch, cut into $1/2$ to 1 inch pieces. If the plant stems are old and woody, strip off leaves and blossoms and bottle only these. Store the bottled dried plant matter in a darkened, cool place, and use as needed.

Catnip will continue to flower throughout its growing season—May through September—and can be harvested more than once during the summer.

Dosages: Use 1 tablespoon of the dried leaves to 1 cup of boiling water. Let steep 10 minutes, remove plant material, and drink three or four times daily. For infant colic, use 1 teaspoon of dried catnip to 1 cup of hot water. Cool to body temperature, remove plant material, and give in a bottle.

To increase the effectiveness of the remedy, add 1 teaspoon of dried fennel seeds (from an herb store, health food store, or your own garden), and steep along with the catnip. Strain, and serve three or four times daily.

CAUTION: Catnip may increase the menstrual flow if taken for cramps. It should therefore be avoided during pregnancy.

FROM THE AUTHOR'S JOURNAL
APRIL 20

Sitting outside on the steps after a hectic morning. The weather is warm—60-ish—and the sun is out. It feels good to just sit and be quiet. A flutter of breeze moves the sumacs, and the scuffling of juncos in the grass is the only sound.

Across from me is the garden. I wander over to see if anything is up yet. In the row for poppies, I find, again, a few green threads. This spring has been so fickle, I could swear they've been up and down several times. Close by, parsley from last year is uncurling wrinkly little fists. In one corner of the plot, chives lift the leaf mulch, and the oregano spreads, twice the size of last year's patch.

Cleaning dead leaves from the oregano, I almost step on another bit of green and peek down to find catnip. Last summer I transplanted catnip at the last minute just as the ground was chilling, but had few hopes for its survival. Now, here it is, just sprouting from the old brown stems. I decide to move the catnip and chives and oregano to a new section of the garden where they won't be harmed when the garden is tilled.

I spend an hour or so digging, sifting out roots of weeds and grass. I pull at sumac roots that are long and orange and rubbery. Stretching as I pull on them, they tear up a tiny path through the soil and finally snap. I pull squishy, purply beet messes left from last year's harvest and toss them into the compost. I save the dandelion babies that come up root and all to use later—the greens for salad and the roots for tea. A few spiders squiggle away. There are lots of earthworms, and I cover them up hoping the robins won't see them.

Finally, the soil is loose and smooth. Chives and parsley and oregano go in next to each other. The catnip gets put at the garden's edge, where it will make a tall border later in the season. I've read, too, that it is a good companion plant for vegetables because the odor repels bugs. We'll see how it works.

As I finish up, I think how nice it is to have a cup of catnip tea, not just when my stomach is upset, but when I'm feeling frazzled. It's cozy and comforting. Last summer, I gathered catnip in a friend's yard, where it grew all around the house like a great fuzzy hedge. This year, I'll be able to get my supply from my own garden. In the meantime, I'll just wait, keeping a watchful eye out for the neighborhood cats and hoping the sun and a little shade from the sumacs will bring me a bountiful harvest.

Experiences with Catnip

A month or so ago, my neighbor called wanting something for her five-year-old son who was running a fever and had symptoms of a cold. I offered catnip to use as a tea, to lower the fever and calm him a bit so he could sleep. Later that day she called to let me know that her son was fine. The fever had broken, and he was up running around, playing again.

And just last week, I gave some of my supply to a friend whose daughter had brought home a new baby. She wanted something for colic, and I told her that catnip, along with an equal amount of fennel seeds, is the best remedy for that problem. Now the baby's doing fine, the mother says, and she keeps catnip and fennel on hand for any future problems.

GOLDTHREAD
Coptis trifolia

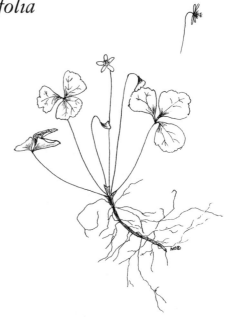

Reflections: Alongside the road, trailing arbutus holds the soil in place. Rain glistens on its leathery leaves and, next to it, tucked into the mosses, is the first goldthread I've seen this spring. Just beyond, a row of trees is marked with bright orange paint— the developer's mark. Mosses here are littered with cigarette butts. A little chill passes through me. Sometime soon this place will disappear, so I stand and soak it up for a little while.

Description: Goldthread is a small, glossy-leaved wildflower found along damp forest floors and in swampy areas where it may form a ground cover and can sometimes be seen to cover entire knolls or fallen logs. The leaves and blossoms look somewhat like wild strawberry.

The leaves are divided into three leaflets and grow from the base of the plant. The leaves are 1–2 inches wide, with a glossy surface, and are evergreen. The leaf edges are slightly scalloped. Leaves spring from a bright gold underground stem that is fine and threadlike: hence the plant's common name. Plant height is up to 6 inches.

Goldthread flowers are white and are composed of five petals that are actually sepals. Blossoms are about $1/2$ inch wide and spring from the base of the plant. They appear on the plant in spring and early summer.

Medicinal Uses: The gold color of goldthread root is due to the chemical berberine, which is intensely bitter. The plant has a few simple uses, and in each case it acts effectively with no apparent side effects. It has been used traditionally as an herbal bitter when appetite and digestion are sluggish or disturbed. It helps to stimulate the digestive juices and prepare the body to break down and assimilate what is eaten. Goldthread can also be used to help heal mouth sores or ulcers, such as cold sores *(Herpes simplex)*. It is a reliable remedy for thrush, an oral yeast infection that affects infants. Used both internally and as an external application, it can help relieve thrush.

Harvesting: Dig the plant up in early spring or in autumn after a frost. Separate the root from the plant, and wash the root carefully. A tincture may be made right away from the fresh root or later from dried root. To dry, cut the roots into small pieces, and spread out on appropriate material. When dried, store for later use.

Dosages: For internal use as an herbal bitter, place 1 tablespoon of fresh or dried root in 1 cup of boiling water, and simmer gently over low heat for 10 minutes. Strain out plant material, and drink about 15 minutes before meals. To use a tincture for the same purpose, place $^1/_4$–$^1/_2$ teaspoon of tincture into a cup of hot water, and drink before meals three times a day.

In cases of thrush, make a tea as directed above. Then soak the tip of a cotton swab in the cooled liquid, and paint the baby's throat carefully and gently several times a day. Three or four drops of the tea may also be mixed in enough water to dilute the taste and given three times a day for the same condition. Nursing mothers may paint their nipples with the wash, or a pacifier may be dipped into the tea and offered to the infant several times a day. For cold sores, a strong tea or the tincture may be applied directly to the affected area several times a day.

Last week I walked into woods I hadn't seen before and found a new path, but it was a workday, with no time for exploring. Today, a Sunday, there is time enough to follow the path as far as it will go.

A light mist falls. Alongside the road, trees are beginning to flower. Mullein puckers from the roadbanks like fuzzy green roses unfolding. Water runs in the ditches and rushes faster in the streams. In the middle of the road, a spotted salamander lies, a woods' sign of wet and early spring. He is as long as my hand, his color as gray and consistent as the wet road. Along his back run two rows of blotchy yellow spots. I move him to a patch of damp brown leaves, and commit him to memory to look up when I get home.

The path juts off the main road, and I walk it for a long time. There are ridges left by truck wheels on either side, but they are old, and leaves and tiny trees in the center are undisturbed. Road sounds disappear. Everything is still. Save for the rain and a few birds, my footsteps are the only sounds. In low places, the path is under water. Leaf litter gives way to muck that is full of animal tracks. Mosses spread beneath the trees so green they seem to glow.

As the rain falls harder, the path becomes a carpet of wintergreen and mosses so thick my feet disappear. Among the bent and brown remains of last year's ferns and blackberry vines that tangle at my legs, I see some goldthread plants. I pluck a few now, clean one root on my jacket, and pop it in my mouth. It's bitter, but not terribly so. A few more go into my pocket, to look at for more details, and to sketch when I get home. The roots of goldthread are so tiny it's hard to imagine harvesting them, but it's good to know they're here if I need them and good to be able to tell them apart from the wild strawberries whose leaves goldthread resembles.

I walk on, and the road where I started appears. Maybe after breakfast I'll go back to gather some goldthread to have on hand. In the meantime, I've seen two treasures in one morning's walk: the spotted salamander, a sign of the season's changing, and goldthread, one of the earth's simple answers to a few old problems.

WHITE PINE
Pinus strobus

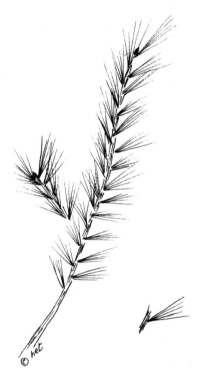

Reflections: The sun is just lifting over the horizon and the air is full of spring smells. Cold gives way to earth and dew scents. Past the barn, smells of cow dung and hay and sweet chimney smoke drift in a breeze. At the development road, on the corner lot, a new row of pine trees has been cut. It looks like a battlefield. So many trees are down, but at least one fallen tree's life will serve some good—the cough medicine I'll make from its inner bark and the joy I have working in the quiet, early day.

Description: Eastern white pine is an evergreen tree bearing 4 to 8 inch narrow cones. The tree is the largest conifer in the Northeast and can reach up to 100 feet in height. It prefers sandy, well-drained soil, and it is often seen in exclusive stands. When growing in dense woods, the trunk of eastern white pine is straight and has horizontal branches that are added at the rate of one row per year of life. In spacious areas where there are no competing trees, the tree may become broad, with trunk divisions and branches that spread wide.

The leaves are evergreen needles 2–5 inches in length, with five needles occurring in each bundle. Although the tree is evergreen, some pale rust-colored needles are shed every fall. Cones are up to 8 inches long, with long stalks and thin, flattened scales that are rounded at the margins. In older trees, the bark is gray and scaly and has furrowed ridges.

Medicinal Uses: White pine bark is an expectorant and respiratory stimulant. It has been used for centuries as a remedy for coughs and chest congestion, including asthma and bronchitis. When used as a base for cough syrups, white pine bark aids expectoration of mucus, thereby helping to prevent worsening of the respiratory symptoms. The bark is also antiseptic and thus helps to reduce or slow down bacterial growth.

Harvesting: The inner bark can be removed from young saplings or narrow branches in the spring. Care should be taken not to remove bark in a complete circle around the tree trunk or branch at any one point, since this type of cut interrupts the flow of nutrients and will cause the death of the tree or branch.

A drawknife is the easiest tool for bark removal, but any sharp knife will do. Cut into the bark, and pull the knife toward you, taking care to lift up just the layer of bark. Grasp the end of bark and pull along the length of branch or trunk. The inner bark is easiest to separate from the outer bark when pieces have begun to dry some. The outer gray bark can be discarded, and the inner living cambium layer spread on screens for drying. After 10 to 14 days, bark should be dry and will snap between your fingers when it is. Bottle and store.

Dosages: Use 1–2 Tablespoons of dried inner bark simmered slowly in 1 cup of water for about 15–20 minutes. Let cool, and drink three or four times daily. Or use the bark strips in a syrup for coughs.

FROM THE AUTHOR'S JOURNAL
APRIL 27

In the hours before work, I am out for a walk, and out to gather white pine bark. Down past Weeks's farm, fallen white pines lay along the new development road where a lot of has been cleared.

The cut trees lie broken and haphazardly stacked. I climb in over a springy network of thin branches, looking for a young, smooth-skinned pine to try. The first tree I come to smells green and fresh, but not piney. Next to it, chopped in sections, are limbs that sparkle with resiny drops. I start shaving from the cut place, and the knife draws back a crusty layer of gray and reddish bark that peels away easily, almost like an avocado skin. Underneath is a fine, fibrous layer that slips away smoothly. And under this layer, a slick of slippery juice coats the wood. I think how like our bodies these trees are, layer covering layer and fluid between the layers, maybe to reduce the friction of growth and movement.

The work is easy. First the gray bark comes off, then my fingers pull at the thin strips of inner bark. I take as many pieces as I can from a section, then move to another. My back gets tired. I stand up to stretch and take a deep breath, and am surprised at how much time has passed.

I could do this work for hours, and maybe I'll come back tonight. For now, time and duty call me home. I pack my pockets with the sticky strips. One fine, pale piece goes into my mouth. It tastes tender and sweet, not the least bit bitter. I chew it like gum, and the walk home smells like a pine forest. Now when I pass the empty rubble lot that used to be woods, I won't be quite so sad. I'll have bits of its wonder tucked away in the cupboard to use once in a while, so the place will heal me still.

Kitchen Notes

At home, I use the pale curls of white pine bark I harvested along with other herbs to make a cough syrup. Out of the cabinet come jars of rose hips and Solomon's seal root and wild cherry bark. I decide to use violets and red clover, too, because they are useful for coughs and chest congestion.

To make the syrup, I snip the pine strips into small bits and put them into a pan—in all, about two large handfuls of the dried curls of bark. Next, I add a handful of rose hips and one of Solomon's seal roots and just a small palmful of wild cherry bark. Together in the pan, the herbs look like a forest floor, full of texture and pale and bright. Over the mixture, I pour golden honey—as much as it takes to cover the herbs. I turn the heat on to medium until the honey liquefies. Then the heat gets turned to low, and the mixture warms and steeps on the stove throughout the day, stirred once in a while.

In the evening, the house smells delightful. I pour off the honey syrup and measure it into a jar. There are bits of bark in it, so I layer cheesecloth over another jar and strain the syrup through. The cheesecloth catches the plant litter, and the syrup that comes through is a dark, rosy brown. I pour it into a clean bottle, label it, and set it in the cabinet to store, knowing it should be good indefinitely because the honey will preserve it. The syrup looks, tastes, and smells so nice, I can't wait to use it.

VIOLET
Viola species

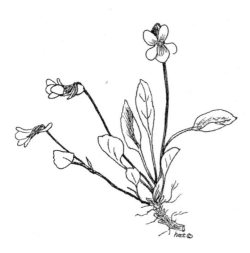

Reflections: A wind blows up the hill, and I look into the woods I came from and at the lake in the distance. The wind whips at me. I am filled with glad affection for this place where there is still room for wild things—for deer who make quiet treks up the hill in the dark, for the hundreds of violets that carpet the spring ground, and for trees and lakes and tiny animals and unbroken winds. If there is ever a time when there are no wild places left for me to go, I'm sure I'll wither away.

Description: The violets are a common spring wildflower, and numerous species occur in our region. Their habitats vary, with some species preferring damp, rich woods and meadows, while others frequent fields and roadsides. The sweet violet, *Viola odorata,* is the violet of herbal tradition, but others may be used in its place with similar results.

Leaves of the species vary in shape, size, and origin of growth. Some plants have only basal leaves, while others have leaves along stems also. In species where leaves occur along stems, the leaves generally grow alternately. Leaves of most species are simple, although in a few, they are deeply lobed. Plant heights vary from 2–15 inches.

Blossoms of most violet species are composed of five petals. The lower petal is generally larger than the rest and has a spur at its base. Color of the blossoms range from white to deep lavender-blue, and some species have yellow blossoms. The flowers of some species are distinctly fragrant, while others have no noticeable scent. Violets may be found in bloom from early spring to early summer.

Medicinal Uses: Violet leaves and blossoms are expectorant and can be used in respiratory congestion to help soften mucus and remove it from the body. A syrup of violets was often used in cough preparations where color and mild taste, along with its action on the respiratory system, made it a good base. Violets can be used to treat mild bronchitis or coughs of influenza and mild colds.

Violets are also considered alterative and work gradually to move the metabolism toward a healthy balance. They have been used as a part of a therapy program for chronic skin conditions, such as eczema and psoriasis. Because of their antiseptic properties, violets have been used externally as a poultice for skin irritations or minor wounds. The leaves and blossoms can be added to a salve for the same problems.

It was thought at one time that violets, as an alterative, were helpful in some cancers, and traditionally violets were thought to be antineoplastic, helping to stop the growth of cancer cells.

Harvesting: Gather the whole plants or just the leaves and blossoms when the plant is just starting to bloom. Spread out to dry on appropriate material. If the whole plants are harvested, turn every day or so to speed thorough drying. When crumbly, store in airtight containers.

Dosages: Make an infusion by pouring 1 cup of boiling water over 1 tablespoon of dried violet leaves and blossoms. Steep for 20 minutes, and then strain out plant parts. Drink three times a day. For skin conditions, crush the fresh plant, and apply directly to the area, or use dried plants in a salve.

An absolutely HOT day! The thermometer reads 75, but I know it's hotter. I decide on a walk, despite the heat, just to see what's growing.

The morning sky is perfect. Along the roadside, birches are fully leafed out. What will become meadow sweet later this season has begun to get green shoots. At the Weeks's farm, the cows are out. This is the final test of spring—when there is enough grass in the fields for the cows to come out of the barn where they have spent 6 or 7 months. So far the cows haven't ventured out of the open gate. They lounge on the hay, soaking up sun they haven't seen for a long time.

Just past the farm, red raspberry vines are leafing out with new green shoots. In some places, the Canada mayflower has taken over, making a green carpet that leads into the woods. Ferns sprout long, pale green arms with a clenched fist of leaflets ready to unfold. I find sweet fern that is just starting to put out its greenish leaves. Even at this early stage, it smells wonderful—heady, deep, spicy. I want to fill my house with it and rub it on my skin and in my hair. I see violets, too, along the roadside, but I won't gather these that grow so close to a road. I do pick a few to press, and then turn down Big Sandy.

I take a path that leads through woods I haven't seen, and decide to follow it. I walk on pine needles and wintergreen. Alongside me, blueberry bushes are full of tiny leaves—such tender green. Flower buds are pink tops on some of them. I lean down to pick a blueberry leaf to chew, and find goldthread in bloom. It seems like only a bit ago that I found the leaves. Spring happens so fast in Maine, everything rushes to get its chance, and I wonder where I've been. I almost missed goldthread in bloom. As I stand up, blackflies dive into my face and hover around my head. Soon, the females will be out, and I'll have to wear netting to come through the woods. Today, a hat will do.

The path I'm following hasn't been used for years, at least not by humans. The soft places are deeply marked with deer prints. Baby balsams close in on both sides. I climb higher and stop at a clearing to look around me. What an amazing place! Mosses of every color and texture cover the open spaces along the edge of the woods. I can see the lake

from here. In the field, the just-coming-up grass is peppered with violets—all different kinds. Large, downy-leaved ones with the dark purple
blossoms, and white ones with maroon veins in the throats, and tiny
paler ones, with small, very round, almost translucent leaves. Every
where I step there are violets.

I sit and pick for a long time. Sit, then slide over a bit, pick more,
slide, pick, slide, until my sack is full of baby violets. When I'm ready to
leave, I walk with the wind up through the fields, past the old garden
where deer have searched through cornstalks, to the road, and home. I
think of how many uses I'll have for my morning's efforts. And I think of
how delightful it will be to have violet tea in the middle of white winter.

Kitchen Notes

On the table next to me is a screen full of violet blossoms, so intensely
purple they are a shock against the plain gray of screen and against this
backdrop of everyday kitchen things. I chew on one small leaf. It tastes
amazing—a neat, clean green.

I decide to try a tincture of violet blossoms just to see what I get. I'm
hoping for lavender-colored tincture. I pour the alcohol over a jarful of
blossoms, and within minutes the liquid is lavender, then deep purple.
My daughter comes in, and we stand looking at the jar as I hold it up in
the sun. An hour later, the alcohol has begun to extract the chlorophyll
from the small green parts that surround each petal, and the tincture is
a pale green. Funny, how some properties break down in the alcohol
faster than others. Maybe next time I'll try it with just the petals. I can't
think of anything lovelier than a violet-colored tincture.

Experiences with Violets

Last year I told a friend about taking violets for coughs. Her children
couldn't stand the yucky taste of some of the stronger herbs, but liked
the idea of using flowers as medicine. They helped their mom with the
harvesting and now each year they'll scour the fields for violets to use
for "flower medicine."

GREATER CELANDINE
Chelidonium majus

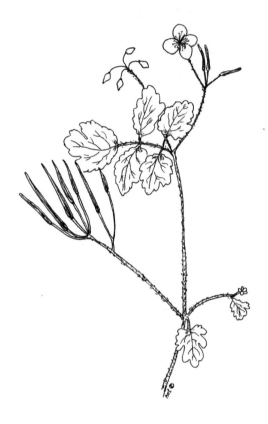

Reflections: In the first of early spring days when fields were full of melting snow, I put on boots and slogged over to the shivering apple trees in the side field to check for deer tracks. There, just barely out of the snow, lay greater celandine, its fancy, pale green leaves clinging to the ground. It's one of my favorite herbs to see, especially under the snows of early spring. It reminds me that the silent earth is just resting and is eager to leap back into life.

Description: Greater celandine is an attractive member of the Poppy family with bright yellow blossoms and decorative leaves that produce a bright yellow-orange latex when torn. It may attain up to 2 feet in height and can be found in damp waste places, along roadsides, and around old building foundations.

The leaves are deeply lobed. On their surface, water beads up in a rain or mist. Leaves may be up to 8 inches in length. When they are torn or crushed, a bright orangey yellow juice is released.

Greater celandine flowers are composed of four regular petals that are deep yellow in color. The blossoms are up to an inch wide and occur in loose clusters at the top of slightly hairy stems. Greater celandine blooms early spring through fall, and both blossoms and seed capsules can often be seen on the same plant. The slender capsules contain many tiny seeds and are 1 to 2 inches in length.

Medicinal Uses: Internally, greater celandine has been used traditionally for inflammations of the gallbladder and for the tendency to form gallstones. The plant is known as a cholagogue and thus stimulates the flow of bile from the gallbladder.

Externally, the juice of the plant is effective in controlling warts and some skin fungi. The fresh juice, applied several times a day, can inhibit the growth or spread of these conditions. It should be used sparingly, however, as it can be caustic to tender skin.

Harvesting: Gather the fresh aerial plant parts when greater celandine is in bloom, and bundle the stem bases to hang for drying. Hang in an airy, shaded place, and store when plant parts are brittle.

Dosages: To use greater celandine as a tea, make a decoction by placing 1 teaspoon of the dried herb in water and bringing it to a boil. Remove from heat, and let steep for 10 minutes. The strained tea can be taken in 1-cup doses three times daily.

To use externally, tear a leaf or the stem, and apply the bright yellow juice to affected skin. A tincture may also be used, or the strong tea used as a wash. Repeat several times daily.

CAUTION: Greater celandine should not be taken during pregnancy. In other cases, the dosages should not be exceeded, as this herb can cause painful purging of the intestines. All parts of the fresh plant are acrid and cause a burning sensation upon taste and contact.

I run my hand through damp hair, wet from the heavy mist that has turned into rain. All the fields are silver with moisture and full of long grasses bent by its weight. Leaves are fully out now. Along roadbanks, ferns are unfolding. Blueberry bushes are packed with flowers—a good year for berries, I think. The violets are still out, and next to them are the blossoms of wild strawberry.

I walk down past the abandoned farmhouse where the porcupines now live. In the winter, little dirty trails through the snow mark their travels. Their low bodies drag a path from tree to barn, from barn to house and back, a telltale sign of the farm's new residents.

I look around now to see if I can spot a porcupine, and notice that the old foundation is crowded with greater celandine in bloom. The plant lines the base of the stone walls and crowds up to the edges of the road. Its lacy leaves are full of silvery rain beads and the flowers are full open—a sun color in this grayish day.

Greater celandine is a lovely and tenacious plant. It weathers sleet and bitter cold, only to spring back again when the sun comes out. It pushes through the asphalt of city parking lots and crowds at the edges of buildings. And near my house, it grows between the stones of a neighbor's front steps. Not much stops its progress. I pluck a bit of leaf now and watch yellow latex pucker at the torn edge. I touch it to my hand, making a pattern of yellow dots, and decide to pick some flowery stems to carry home, even though this herb still scares me a little. I know it can be dangerous if taken in too-large doses, and I've only used it a few times. Already I can feel the tender skin between my fingers start to burn where the yellow juice has smeared. Maybe if I dry the plant and use it as a tea, it will be less acrid.

Still, I'll always be cautious with this herb. It reminds me of how tentative the line between healing and harm can be. I start for home with my celandine, and the mist turns into real rain. The water makes little rivers through my hair, tickling.

Kitchen Notes

At home, I bundle some of the celandine to dry. The intense color of its blossoms lights up the room, and I remember my first summer in Maine when I gathered greater celandine from around the barn. It grew there like a bright, sunny ring around the building, right next to the yellow buttercups. Now, with some of the remaining plants, I decide to make a fresh-plant tincture. I cut small pieces into a jar and pour alcohol over them. Yellow color leaches out into the liquid right away, and I set the jar in a cupboard. A few weeks later the color has deepened into a dark orange. The inside of the bottle is coated, and while the tincture is clear, the latex clings so tenaciously to the glass I have to shake the bottle to see the liquid. I am reminded again of this herb's strength and of the care I have to take when using it.

ELDERBERRY
Sambucus canadensis and *pubens*

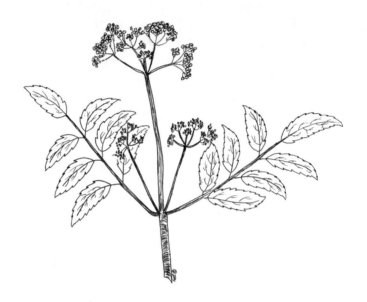

Reflections: Today, the elderberry blossoms are dropping from the bush in any breeze. It's time to gather them before it's too late, and wind and time take them away. A fat bumblebee is annoyed. He knows this bounty is his, not mine, and he guards his property suspiciously, circling my hat. I am courteous and move out of his way to pick in another place. My hand grows yellow-green with pollen and the bumblebee gives up, allowing me to share this season's riches. In my basket, elder blossoms pile like fluffy clouds.

Description: The elderberries are tall, woody-stemmed shrubs that bear profuse white or ivory blossoms and are common to moist thickets and along roadsides. The elders are found in moist soils, and the red-berried variety is often found in rocky areas. Two species of elder are used interchangeably for medicinal purposes. The common elder, *Sambucus canadensis,* bears tart, edible purplish black berries that are often used in making wild jams and jellies. The red-berried elder, *Sambucus pubens,* produces very acrid-tasting red berries that are known to be somewhat toxic, causing digestive upsets.

The leaves in both species are divided and sharply toothed and are opposite. Each divided leaf is composed of five to eleven leaflets in the common elder and five to seven in the red-berried elder. All leaflets are lance- or egg-shaped and are sharply pointed.

In the common elder, flowers are tiny five-lobed blossoms that are up to $\frac{1}{6}$ inch wide and are fragrant. They occur in a flattened cluster at the ends of leafy branches. Clusters are from 2 to 10 inches wide. In the red-berried variety, flowers are fragrant, $\frac{1}{4}$ inch wide, with five petals, and are white or ivory in color. They occur in tall, roughly tri-angular clusters atop terminal branches. The red-berried variety can be found in bloom first—in spring through early summer. Common elder blooms about a week or so later—in early summer.

The fruit in both species is a juicy berry. In the common elder, fruits appear in flat-topped clusters of purplish black berries, while in the red-berried species, red berries grow in pyramid-shaped clusters.

Medicinal Uses: The blossoms of both species can be used as a tea to help lower fever. The herb is diaphoretic, producing a sweat and thereby allowing the body to be cooled in a natural way. A tea of el-derberry blossoms is useful for treating colds or flu with accompany-ing fever. The herb is especially nice to use for children, as it makes a tasty tea that works gently. The flowers can also be used for hay fever or sinusitis, because they help lower the reactivity of mucous mem-branes to allergens.

Harvesting: Gather blossoms by cutting or breaking off the whole cluster at the stem. Spread the clusters out on screens or baskets in a shaded place where there is good air circulation. Remove the blos-soms from the stems when they are dried, and store.

Dosages: Use 1 tablespoon of dried blossoms to 1 cup of boiling water for an infusion. Allow to steep for 10–20 minutes, strain out plant material, and take three times a day. Elder flowers can also be taken in a half-and-half mixture with either yarrow or peppermint, both of which are mild tasting and have the same diaphoretic effect. This mixture is especially nice for children.

CAUTION: Any temperature over 100 degrees, or a fever that lasts more than a few hours, should be attended to by a licensed physician.

FROM THE AUTHOR'S JOURNAL
MAY 29

Today is the first sunny day after a week of clouds and rain and mist, and I am tackling the lawn. Because the sun is out, so are the black flies, and I race around the yard in a hat and long sleeves and long-legged pants. I mow in a frenzy, then dash inside for a moment's peace. I take off my hat and notice the dusting of pollen where I have streaked back and forth beneath the elderberry bushes, and it reminds me that the blossoms are opening and ready to harvest.

I walk out to the elderberry bushes near the barn and break off a first flower cluster. When I pick it, tiny flowers nearby fall to the ground. I decide to use a basket to catch them, to save whatever flowers fall. The work is slow, and I try shaking the clusters over my basket to catch just the flowers. But when I shake one cluster, others beyond the basket drop their flowers too.

I resort to picking the whole, individual clusters one by one and laying them gently in the basket. Soon, the flowery clusters pile high and look so pretty I wish I had my camera to take a picture. My hands grow polleny, and I rub at them to get rid of the yellow stuff, but it just spreads over my skin, softening it like a talc.

When the basket is full, I am surprised to see that the bush is still loaded with blossoms. There are lots left to form berries for the birds who will enjoy them and lots left for the fat bumblebee who claimed the bush as his but let me share the bounty.

I pick one more perfect flower cluster to press and label. This bush is the red-berried elder, *Sambucus pubens.* Next to it stands the "official" plant, *Sambucus canadensis,* or common elder. It is just beginning to bud. Soon there will be blossoms and this flowery work will start all over again. Which is just fine with me.

Kitchen Notes

To prepare the elderberry for drying, I sit at the table and pluck each flower from its tiny stem. I pull the clusters through my hands, making little rakes of my fingers. The blossoms smell funny-sweet, a little fruity, and very polleny.

After half an hour or so, I'm all finished. Every tiny cream-colored flower is separated from its thin white stem. I scoop them up in my hands and bury my face in them sniffing. I spread some of them out on screens to dry for tea, and the rest go in a jar with alcohol over them to make tincture. The pollen on my hands feels so good I rub it all over my arms to soothe my skin. I clean up the table, scooping up bits and pieces of elderberry stems and leaves to go back under the bushes. They can make compost, feeding the plants for next year's crop.

Experiences with Elderberry

Last year's supply of elderberry flowers went to friends for fevers, especially for their children. It made a nice, good-tasting tea, with no bitterness. I dried lots to have on hand and used the tincture in formulas for flu and colds to help break fevers.

CLEAVERS
Galium aparine

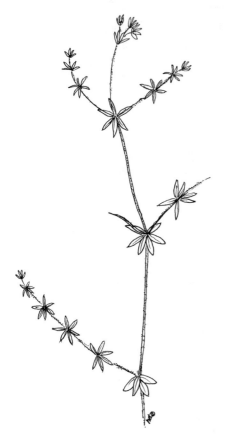

Reflections: In the woods everything is quiet. Each time I come here it feels like such a change from the sunny, busy field. At the clearing where the tiny stream bubbles down a hill, growth is lush, and the water is mostly hidden by cleavers that bunch along the stream-bed. Everything in me slows, stills, and I stop for a moment and take a deep breath before moving on.

Description: Cleavers is a weak-stemmed wildflower often found reclining on or vining about neighboring plants. Single stems of cleavers may grow up to 6 feet in length if uncut, and the plant may be found in thick mats on the ground if there is nothing nearby on which they can climb. The plant is somewhat juicy when picked. It grows in woods and thickets and is often found near moist ground.

The stem of cleavers is squared and covered with hooked bristles that allow the plant to cling to anything around it. The plant is a member of the Bedstraw family, and of the several species that look alike, none but cleavers has bristles.

The leaves grow up to 3 inches long and occur in whorls of six to eight along the square stem. The simple leaves are lance shaped, with pointed tips, and they, like the stem, are covered with bristles.

Cleavers blossoms are tiny, about $^1/_8$ inch wide, and have four petals. The blossoms occur in loose clusters that spring from leaf axils. Flowering time is early to mid-summer, May through July or August.

Medicinal Uses: Internally, cleavers is useful in problems of the urinary tract, where it acts as a diuretic and an anti-inflammatory. It can be used as a tea in bladder infections and for painful urination. Cleavers has also been used for relief of water retention, such as premenstrual edema. It can be helpful in persons with a tendency to form kidney stones or gravel and, in this case, is best as a fresh-plant tincture, or as a juice, if a juicer is available.

Cleavers is also alterative and tonic, toning the body generally and altering metabolism toward a healthful balance. It has been used in chronic skin conditions, such as psoriasis, where it aids in elimination of toxins from the body. As an alterative, cleavers works on the lymphatic system, and it can be a useful adjunct in therapies for swollen lymph glands and any associated problems, such as tonsillitis or mononucleosis.

Externally, cleavers can be used as a wash or salve for burns or wounds.

Harvesting: The aerial parts of the plant are used. Cut or break off the stems at ground level when they are green and healthy looking, and bundle loosely. Cleavers will actually bundle itself, as it clings to everything, and you need not tie it together with rubber bands. Examine the plant material carefully for insects or rotted plant parts, and then spread it out loosely on screens, baskets, or drying racks. Cleavers dries fairly rapidly and should be crumbly before it is stored. A fresh-plant tincture may be made soon after gathering by chopping the herb into small bits and covering it with alcohol or vinegar in a jar.

Dosages: Use 1–2 tablespoons of the dried herb to 1 cup of boiling water, and let steep for 10–20 minutes. This tea can be drunk three times a day. For kidney stones or gravel, the fresh-plant tincture can be taken in doses of 2 teaspoons three times daily, or the fresh juice can be used, if you can express it, in the same dosages.

Externally, simply crush the fresh plant, and apply to the skin. The plant material may be held in place by a bandage or gauze. The dried plant can also be used in an ointment or salve for skin problems.

FROM THE AUTHOR'S JOURNAL
JUNE 8

From this window, I can see out to the garden where one scarlet poppy—our first bloom—has opened with the sun. At the bird feeder, purple finches and blue jays and goldfinches are breakfasting. It is 6 AM, and already this morning I've been out to the garden to say hello to the new poppy and look at the beginnings of corn in the back garden. I picked off a few slugs sneaking up on the sage, and now I'm off to gather cleavers.

The long grass in the back field has not been mowed yet, and lots of dogbane stands with its dainty folded leaves, looking pretty and buying time before the mower comes. Down the piney path into the woods, greenery is pushing up through the pine needle litter. St. John's-wort is tall now in this transition zone where field becomes forest, but it has no hint of blossoms forming.

Farther down the path to the stream, pyrola is green and lush and creeps out to cover the walkway. I stop to look at its round leaves and check for a flower spike starting, but find none yet. Sometime this summer I'll gather this plant too, but this morning I've got something else in mind. Down near the water, I find the cleavers I'm looking for, so tall and heavy the knot of plants lean over onto the grasses surrounding the streambed.

I start gathering, picking handfuls at a time. The stems are 2 or 3 feet long. And they cling to each other, making their own bundle. As I touch the leaves and stems that are roughened with tiny sand-papery bumps, I remember all the cat-baths I have had, given by cat friends with rough and loving tongues that scraped away at my skin. Cleavers feels like that—like little cat tongues working at me.

Pieces of the plant dangle from my sleeves as I work. They attach themselves, and I have to pull them off to add them to the bundle. Some of the plants come up root and all. I try to be careful, but the roots are shallow, and some whole plants come up anyway. They smell like earth and water, and I press my nose into the scratchy mass and sniff long and deep.

When I've gathered all that I can for today, I pick long grass sprigs and a fat yellow slug from the bundle. I walk farther down the path to peek at the lady's slippers again, then turn around for home.

Kitchen Notes

In the herb room, cleavers hang from the old collapsible clothes dryer on the wall. The spread-out slats make a green, hairy fan we have to walk around, and the whole room smells deep and earthy. I pop a piece of leaf into my mouth and chew. It feels funny. It doesn't collapse and disappear like a simple leaf might, but sort of bites back. I remember wondering how frogs feel when they swallow live ants and decide that now I know. Even after I swallow, my throat feels the prickles.

This batch of cleavers is drying to use sometime later in tea, along with other herbs, for bladder infections. I heard recently that cleavers can be used to treat kidney stones, too, but that the fresh plant is best for that. I wonder if a fresh-plant tincture would work, and I decide to go back and gather another batch of cleavers to try that way. It always amazes me how much I don't know. But learning is so much fun, it doesn't matter.

SHINLEAF
Pyrola elliptica and species

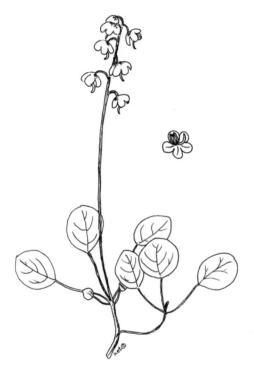

Reflections: The air along the road-side smells like watermelon—fresh and juicy. Every breath is a balm for my frazzled soul that has been caught up in too many things lately. When I enter the woods, the path is cool and shadowy. Not much light has slipped in here. My eyes are glued to the forest floor, watching for shinleaf. I find it and taste a leaf. It leaves a bitterness on my tongue and a deeper, fruity un-dertaste—a good taste first thing in this new day.

Description: Shinleaf is a small, perennial, evergreen member of the Wintergreen family found in woodlands. A number of *Pyrola* species grow in our area, and all have roughly the same chemical components. The plants are generally found in woodlands, either dry or moist.

For most species, leaves are generally round or oval shaped and basal. Leaf length is up to 3 inches, but may be smaller in some species. In shinleaf, *Pyrola elliptica,* leaves are oval or oblong and dark green, with a reddish leaf stalk. In the round-leaved pyrola, *Pyrola americana*, leaves are quite round and are tough and leathery, with a shiny surface. Leaves of most species have slight, irregular toothing. Plant heights range from 2 to 10 inches.

Shinleaf flowers occur on a central spike. In general, they are about $^1/2$ inch wide and are white with pinkish or greenish tints. The blossom has five petals and ten stamens and a style that is conspicuous as it protrudes much beyond the petals. Flowers occur early summer through fall. Generally, the pyrolas are small insignificant-looking plants and are easy to miss unless in flower.

Fruit occurs as a four- or five-chambered seed capsule, roundish in shape, along the central stem. The capsule remains on the plant even into the next spring sometimes.

Medicinal Uses: All the pyrolas share similar chemical constituents. They are strongly astringent, antiseptic, diuretic, and analgesic, and they contain salicin, the basic compound in aspirin.

Traditionally, *Pyrola elliptica* was known as shinleaf because early settlers and Native Americans used a poultice of the freshly crushed leaves for recent bruises and sprains, to relieve pain and inflammation.

Because of their astringent, diuretic, and antiseptic properties, the pyrolas are useful in urinary tract infections, where they will increase the flow of urine and aid in eliminating toxins from the body. Pyrola can also be helpful in PMS, where urinary tract infections accompany the menstrual cycle.

Harvesting: The aerial parts are gathered any time during the growing season, although it is preferable to gather the plants when they are in bloom. If enough stem material is available, bundle in small batches and hang to dry. Otherwise, simply spread the plants out along screens or in baskets out of the sun. Some species with leathery leaves may take longer to dry than the thin-leaved varieties, so check thoroughly for dryness before storing.

Dosages: For tea, pour 1 cup of boiling water over 1 tablespoon of the crushed dried leaves, and let steep for 20–30 minutes. In the thicker-leaved varieties, the leaves can be simmered over low heat for 10 minutes instead. Drink 1 cup of tea three times daily. If taking the tincture as opposed to the tea, use 15–30 drops three times daily.

CAUTION: People with allergies or sensitivities to aspirin products should probably avoid using this herb.

FROM THE AUTHOR'S JOURNAL
JUNE 9

A crescent moon is up in the eastern sky that is mottled with slate and orange. In a nearby tree some unknown bird makes a funny call, and in the maple, one starling chatters. A goldfinch darts across the back field—a flash of bright yellow bobbing—and mourning doves coo at me from the sumacs.

I take slow and deep breaths, tasting again a violet leaf chewed awhile ago, and decide to walk down to the woods where I ski sometimes in the winter. The last time I was there, about a month ago, I was out to pick violets. Along the way, I saw a large stand of pyrola, and that's what I'm after today. I've never come upon it in full bloom, but if it's flowering, I'll be able to gather some to tincture.

I walk down past the overgrown field, past a stone wall, and into the woods that are still full of shadows. Along the forest floor, low blueberry bushes are starting to set fruit. Flowers have dropped off and little green swellings are visible. Canada mayflower is here, too, ever present, and lady's slipper leaves are full and ribbed.

I stop at a stone wall that breaks for this path and discover a matrix of walls that intersect and divide these woods that must have once been pasture. The stones are covered with a fur of old pine needles and moss, and the wall where I stand looks like a great sleeping dragon. At its base is the stand of pyrola clustered along the woods floor. The leaves are bright and round, and each plant has a flower spike with blooms along its length. I've seen the old brown stems of flowers in late fall, and even now, they stand next to this season's new plants. The flowers are unusual, and more whitish than the pink I expected, but beautiful. I kneel to gather some of the plants to take home.

As I pick, whole plants come up. The roots are strung together on runners, so when I pick one plant, I disturb its neighbors and have to be careful. As I pull plants up, litter from the forest floor clings to their roots and lower leaves. Pine needles and humusy soil and translucent hardwood leaves all have to be plucked out bit by bit. It's good work, though—so focused and earthy that everything else disappears. There is just this one plant, this one tiny root, this one leaf tangled in rusty pine needles. There is just this bit of earth to be shaken out and brushed away, just these shiny leaves to be checked and cleaned, and this one bag to be filled. I become this peaceful work, and everything else disappears.

Kitchen Notes

At home, I rinse out humus from the roots and rinse the plant leaves too. Then I chop the pyrola into a jar and cover it with grain alcohol. It goes into the herb cabinet next to the chickweed and comfrey tinctures that are in the making, too. The table is full of the droppings of my work: rusty pine needles and bits of humus, a few pyrola leaves, and some greenish white petals from its flowers. I brush them together and scoop them up for the compost pile. A tiny inchworm waves at the air from one leaf edge, looking for something familiar. He gets transplanted to the irises by the dooryard steps and slips away.

Outside, one fat, pinkish mourning dove stands at the edge of the hanging birdbath and watches a chipmunk scavenge in the daylilies. The sun lights up the wet fields and grass. Bits of white fluff move along the new blue sky. I chew a last pyrola leaf and get ready for the day.

CHICKWEED
Stellaria media and species

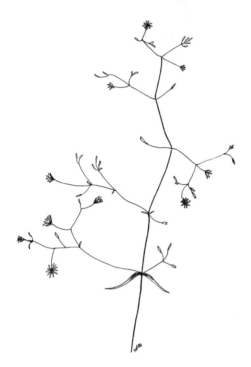

Reflections: The fields these days are full of life—spittlebugs, and bees, and dragonflies thrive in and just above the lush green. In the apple trees out back, bobolinks are nesting and the air smells fresh and sweet with growing things. I find a patch of chickweed, where dainty, starry flowers lean on slender stems against their neighbors. The mosquitoes surround me like a halo, but I am undeterred and work until I have a full harvest and a little more wisdom to use throughout the year.

Description: This weak-stemmed, recumbent wildflower is found in fields, lawns, and waste places. It grows as individual plants, but appears in puffy, tangled mats. The numerous varieties of *Stellaria,* known as chickweed, may be used interchangeably with similar results. *Stellaria media* is the official herb of traditional medicinal use. It is edible as well as medicinal and is eaten as a tasty spring and summer green, boiled or steamed for a short time.

Leaves in *Stellaria media* are up to 1 inch long and occur in opposing pairs. They are oval shaped and have smooth margins. The stems are highly branched, and they are marked with a line of tiny hairs along the length, with the line of hairs alternating sides after each leaf pair. Individual plants may grow up to 1¹/₂ feet in height, but since the plant is usually found reclining on neighboring plants, it appears shorter.

The flowers are white, up to ¹/₄ inch wide, with five petals that are so deeply divided there appear to be ten petals. Blossoms appear May through July, and occur in small clusters at the ends of top branches, or they may grow from the leaf axils.

Medicinal Uses: Chickweed has a number of uses. It is emollient and vulnerary, working to soften skin and help in healing skin irritations. It is useful externally in minor wounds and itching. It can be used as a wash, poultice, or salve with good results, or it can be added to other herbs for the same purpose.

Internally, chickweed is somewhat alterative and anti-inflammatory. It is also mildly diuretic and laxative. These properties in combination make it a good adjunct in natural therapies for arthritis, rheumatism, or other chronic inflammatory processes, where it can help in altering metabolism while aiding the body in breaking down and eliminating toxins.

Because of its diuretic and alterative properties, chickweed can be helpful in mild fevers. As a diuretic and laxative, the herb has traditionally been added to formulas for weight control.

Harvesting: Gather the aerial plant parts when the plant is coming into flower. The individual stems can be bundled at their bases and held together with a rubber band. Or the plant can simply be dried by spreading it on screens or baskets. The plant dries easily and should be ready to store in about 10 days. If you will not be using all the chickweed you have harvested, it can be tinctured to assure its stability.

Dosages: Chickweed is tasty as a tea. Its properties are water soluble and are released in boiling water. For internal use, place 2 tablespoons of dried herb in a cup, and pour boiling water over it. Let steep 15–20 minutes and drink three or four times daily. Use 50–60 drops of the tincture three or four times daily.

For external use, make a poultice by crushing the fresh plant and applying it directly to cleaned minor wounds. Or pour a bit of boiling water over the fresh plant, let sit for a few minutes, and then apply the limp plant material to the area. Hold the plant material in place with gauze, and change often. The gauze may be further moistened with the water used to pour over the plant.

A salve can be made for minor wounds, itching, or skin irritations, using chickweed alone or in combination with other herbs.

FROM THE AUTHOR'S JOURNAL
JUNE 11

This morning I'm in the field to pick chickweed. The long grasses are topped with red or silver flower fluff and blow in the breeze, making waves. Purple vetch, orange hawkweed, creamy yarrow, and golden buttercups are all blooming. In some places, the grass is matted flat where deer have slept.

Trying to find an easy place to work, I follow an animal trail to a patch of ground where the grasses are only thigh high. Dew and the white foam of spittlebugs dampen my pants and shoes. Mosquitoes are active already, and fat flies with dappled wings dive-bomb at me. I find a place where chickweed forms a tangle, and start picking.

It's hard from high up to separate the chickweed from the grasses, so I squat to the plant's level to see if that helps. Gathering chickweed is not as easy as I expected. The stem is so thin and limp it tangles in the long grasses, and I keep breaking off just the top flowery bits when it is the whole plant I want. This work takes time and attention, but I'm impatient. My hands are full of spittlebug drool. The mosquitoes have found my fingers and already I can feel them itching with unseen bites. I've picked two ticks off my pants, and my bag is filling much too slowly. In the midst of grumbling to myself about such tedious work, the sun makes it up over a ridge and warms my face with a little kiss. I forget all the trouble with chickweed. Maybe chickweed isn't the problem. Maybe it's me and my hurry-scurry thinking. I give up and just pick for a while, trying a new method. Instead of focusing on the flowers, I look deep into the grass to spot the chickweed stem. It's easy to tell from the grass, with its pair of leaves here and there. So I aim for that, and it works out fine. I pull up the stem near the base and the rest of the plant follows. Soon my bag is full. I gather a bouquet of purple vetch and buttercups, and walk home in the early sun.

Kitchen Notes

At home, I spread some of the chickweed out to dry. Starry little blossoms prop up in a nest of bright green stems. I decide to make a fresh-plant tincture, too, to use in formulas along with other herbs. I chop the skinny stems and blossoms and pack them in a jar, then cover them with alcohol. As I work, I think about all the things I'll do with the herb I've gathered today: chickweed for reducing fevers and water buildup, chickweed as a skin dressing, chickweed as a laxative, chickweed as a food. So many uses! I clean up the plant scraps and pat the herb in place on the drying baskets. For all the complaining I did earlier, there is a full harvest of chickweed drying, and a jar of tincture making—a good day's work!

SUMMER

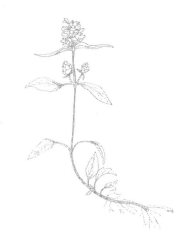

PLANTAIN
Plantago species

Reflections: All the color has dwindled from the summer sky, and soon the bats will start gliding out from under the eaves. I can't make myself go inside. Wind blows at my hair and clothes, whipping them around me. I wish I could stay up all night and watch everything change. I wish I could just lie in the plantain like the deer and watch the night world move softly by.

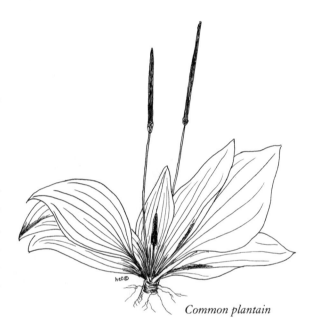

Common plantain

Description: The plantains vary somewhat in size and leaf shape, but share basic characteristics that make identification fairly simple. All of the plantains have only basal leaves, which sprout out from the root and occur in a whorl at ground level. The leaves of all plantain species have deep parallel veins, and when torn, exhibit strong fibers that pull out from the leaves, much like rubbery threads. Plantains are common and abundant, growing in lawns, fields, along roadsides, and in disturbed areas. They can get very large where soil is moist.

The common plantain, *Plantago major,* has broad oval-shaped leaves that grow from to 6 to 8 inches long and 4 inches wide. The leaves are smooth edged. The flowers are tiny and are crowded along a long central spike that erupts from the basal leaves. Fruit, which forms along the flower spike, consists of small brownish seed capsules. Plant height can be up to 18 inches.

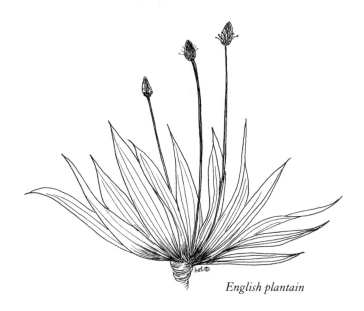

English plantain

The English plantain, *Plantago lanceolata,* has long, narrow, lance-shaped leaves that can grow up to 16 inches in length. This species has a central flower spike covered with tiny indistinguishable flowers, followed by seeds.

Medicinal Uses: Plantain's primary medicinal value is its astringent quality. The fresh, crushed leaf will help reduce inflammation in insect bites or stings. Fresh bruised leaves can also be laid inside a baby's diaper for mild diaper rashes. A dried tea of plantain can be used for mild diarrhea, and the dried plant can be used in salves for hemorrhoids.

The whole plant, leaves and root, are demulcent and expectorant, and a tea of the dried plant can be helpful in coughs and chronic lung conditions, such as asthma or bronchitis, where it will soothe irritated membranes and promote expectoration of mucus. The dried seeds can be used as a bulk laxative.

Harvesting: Fresh leaves can be picked when they are needed from early spring through the beginning of winter when snow covers the ground. Cut leaves from the plant at its base, or pull up whole plants. Dry the plant material on screens, in baskets, or on paper, turning every day or so to allow proper circulation. Once dry, store properly for later use.

To gather seeds, cut flower spikes when seeds are dark and crumble easily. Bundle seed stalks at the bases with rubber bands and hang to dry for 1 or 2 weeks. To store, strip seeds off spikes, and place in a lidded jar.

Dosages: To use externally for insect bites, simply chew or crush the fresh leaf and apply directly to the skin. Use a bandage if desired to keep the leaf in place. An ointment or salve made with the dried leaves can be applied frequently to insect bites or hemorrhoids. For internal use as a tea, add 1 teaspoon of dried leaves to 1 cup of boiling water, steep, strain, and take three or four times daily for diarrhea or for coughs and chronic respiratory problems.

For a bulk laxative, place 1–2 tablespoons of dried seeds into warm water, let sit for 10–15 minutes, then stir, and drink the mixture.

FROM THE AUTHOR'S JOURNAL
JUNE 12

The sun is going down, but there is still lots of light. A few birds talk in the trees. A few blackflies nag at me. A little breeze stirs. It's a wonderful evening, full of fresh and cooling air.

This day was full of earthy chores that lie half done around me now. In the side yard, chicken wire is spread out waiting to be put up for the sweet peas to lean against. Out in the garden, snow peas are trellised on slats and string. In the middle of the front yard, the lawn-mower makes one flame-colored spot in a sea of green. And against the steps, blue flag waits to be divided, bruise-colored buds barely hidden in the leafy sheaths.

The newly cut grass is soft and feels good to walk through barefoot. In the places that haven't been mown yet, plantain stands tall. Its flower stalks have come lately, full of pale white fluff. Before tomorrow, before cutting the rest of the yard, I decide to gather some of its leaves for salve and for tea.

I squat down and grab a leaf at its base and pull. The leaf stretches a bit, then gives. Stringy fibers of the long parallel veins rip away. I pick from one clump, then switch to another and pick more. The flat, shiny leaves are cool beneath my feet. Before long, I have an apron full of plantain, and I sit back down at the dooryard steps to watch the sunset.

The light bleeds from the sky, and the air and trees and grass are all the same shade of greenish gray. A breeze has ripened into wind. The blue flag shifts against the steps, and the leaves of the maple tree are rustling. From the back field come the voices of a thousand new crickets, singing the night to sleep. The air smells sweet, full of mown grass and the new-green scent of fresh plantain in my lap. I wish there weren't chores and Monday nagging. But at least there is plantain, with flowery stalks bending in the wind.

Experiences with Plantain

Last year I made a salve of plantain and other herbs to use for insect bites, and it worked fine. The swelling stayed down, and the bites didn't itch as much. Mostly, though, we used plantain fresh, wadded up and taped over beestings we received walking barefoot through the grass. Nice, that it grew so close to where we needed it.

YARROW
Achillea millifolium

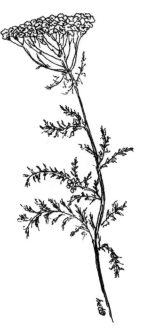

Reflections: These summer days when I walk, I don't go out with any herb in mind to gather. There is such abundance, I never have to decide. Something always presents itself. This morning there is yarrow, standing along the roadsides in full bloom, and in the fields where it is tucked into the tall grasses, its flowers are just starting to open. It is such a pretty plant, so feathery and graceful, I want to take some home and grow it in the garden just for fun.

Description: Yarrow is a common and attractive wildflower of road-sides, fields, and waste places. Many varieties of yarrow have been cultivated for ornamental purposes. The wildflower is a perennial and is rather undemanding as to soil type or moisture. It is a good candidate for cultivation in wildflower gardens and often makes its way into wildflower bouquets.

The leaves of yarrow are distinctive. They are very finely divided with a feathery appearance and feel. The leaves are up to 8 inches long on the lower part of the plant and get smaller as they ascend the stem. Leaves of first-year or young plants can often be seen poking out of the ground with no flower stems visible. On mature plants, leaves occur alternately, are stalkless, and appear grayish green in color. The stem is the same dusky green color and is often covered with white down. Upon crushing, the leaves and stem give off a strong scent. The plants may attain a height of 3 feet.

Yarrow flowers are creamy white and very small, with five petals surrounding a tiny central disk. The blossom is up to $1/4$ inch wide, and flowers occur in a flattened cluster, or corymb, atop the single stem. Yarrow may be found in bloom early summer through fall.

Medicinal Uses: The aerial parts of yarrow have a number of medicinal properties. It is diaphoretic, antipyretic, and anti-inflammatory. These properties make it useful in treating colds and flus where it will promote sweating, help control fever, and reduce inflammatory reactions. With mild expectorant properties, yarrow can also aid in ridding the body of mucus produced with a respiratory infection.

Yarrow is hemostatic and antiseptic and can be useful for treating minor skin wounds or abrasions. The crushed flowers or leaves can be applied externally to clean cuts, where it should help stop bleeding and prevent infection. Yarrow is diuretic to some extent, and this quality added to its hemostatic and antiseptic properties make it helpful in treating mild bladder irritations or infections. In this case, yarrow helps to increase urine flow, while reducing bacteria and controlling bleeding that accompanies the condition.

As a hemostatic and emmenagogue, the herb can be used for excessive menstrual bleeding. Yarrow is also carminative and makes a sensible remedy for mild stomach upsets.

Harvesting: Cut the stems a few inches above the ground just as yarrow comes into flower, and bundle them with rubber bands. Hang to dry, and store when crumbly to the touch. Remove the flowers and leaves, and use these and thinner stem parts, discarding the woody stems.

Dosages: The medicinal properties of yarrow are water soluble, and it makes an effective tea. Use 1 tablespoon of dried herb to 1 cup of boiling water. Steep for 10–20 minutes, and drink three times a day.

I sit at the dooryard steps, and the sky is just as it was last night when I made myself go in, full of the pale greenish gray that brings no color to anything. Except that in the east, orange slides up at the horizon, and second by second, there is more light. A breeze blows and feels good after yesterday's suffocating heat. Today is hotter than yesterday already. The season seems to be racing ahead of itself. Despite its sudden fierceness, I'm glad summer is here. The herbs are coming up so fast it's hard to keep up with them. I go for a walk to see what's new.

In the front yard, one blue flag bud is unsheathed and ready to open, and across the road, a stand is blooming already. I check along the stone wall for what I think is tansy, escaped from a garden years ago. Today the plants are still not showing any blooms but I'm glad to see them anyway. Later in the season, I will harvest some.

Just down the road at Weeks's farm I see what I think is a cat, moving slowly. Then I realize it is a porcupine, the first I've seen up close. It walks with a swaying motion, as if the full backside of bristles is hard to manage. I walk closer slowly, and the porcupine stops and raises its quills some. I squat nearby and just look. This animal must not be fully concerned because it raises its quills only a bit, and then shifts off around the house toward a protective cover of ferns. Once away from me, she runs, swaying side to side. I get up and decide to walk down Big Sandy. A few bugs nag at me, but mostly things are quiet.

Around the field that borders the sloping road, a stone wall stands. Tall grasses rise up around its base, and floating in the sea of green stands yarrow—one of my first herb friends. I climb over the wall and squat to gather some. Seeing it in bloom now, I remember all the years when the kids were young and helped me pick yarrow to use for tea. It's an old standby at our house, and every year I gather some to have on hand. I pluck a leaf now that tastes a little bitter as I chew it. Yarrow has a scent, too, that I always recognize—hard to describe but familiar. I pick for a while in the increasing heat, until the mosquitoes drive me home. But I have treasures—a bundle of yarrow to dry and porcupines to look up and learn more about. There is tansy to keep an eye on, and a morning full of wonder to recall.

Kitchen Notes

At home, I separate the yarrow into small batches, and gather the stem bases in rubber bands. The bundles get hung to dry from the herb rack in the middle of the room, and soon the house fills with the sweet strange scent. Out in the lawn, leaves of first-year yarrow decorate the grass, low feathery clusters of bright, light green, promising another harvest before season's end.

Experiences with Yarrow

Last year I offered a tea of yarrow to a woman with a bladder infection. It helped stop the mild bleeding she was having, and made urinating less painful for her. In just a few days, the infection had cleared up and she was back to normal. And just a few months ago, when the flu season hit our house, we used yarrow along with peppermint in a tea to help control the fever. It tasted fine, and worked—such gentle and sure results from such an easy herb!

RED CLOVER
Trifolium pratense

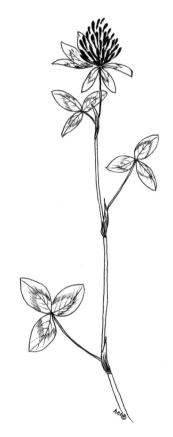

Reflections: I like this hand-picking of clover. It is like a meditation, so focused and repetitive. When I look around me, there is more red clover than when I started. It reminds me of the loaves and fishes story—the more I use, the more there is. It makes me want to leap and sing with gratitude.

Description: Red clover is a tall clover that grows upright to 2 feet in height. It can be found in old fields and lawns, along roadsides, and in waste places where soil has been disturbed. It will tolerate some shade, but prefers full sun. Red clover is sometimes planted as a green manure to improve soil, since it helps fix nitrogen in the soil when turned under. Adequate rain encourages lush growth, but red clover can survive droughty conditions to some extent, although the flower heads tend to dry out more quickly if the soil is dry. The plant flowers from May through September throughout the United States and will come back after being mowed to produce more blossoms if allowed.

Red clover leaves are divided into 3 leaflets that are oval shaped and blunt-tipped. The leaves are $1/2$ to 2 inches long, and each bears a pale V-shaped blotch on its surface.

The individual flowers are tiny and shaped much like the blossom of the common garden pea. Flowers are clustered in dense heads atop erect, finely hairy stems. The color ranges from pinkish lavender to reddish magenta. Flower heads are about 1 inch long, and $1/2$ to 1 inch wide. As flowers fade, they turn a rusty brownish color around the edges and begin to appear dried and bedraggled.

Medicinal Uses: The dried flower heads of red clover are known to be expectorant, antispasmodic, alterative, and antitussive. These qualities make it useful for soothing coughs and chest congestion, where it will inhibit coughing, promote the flow of mucus, and act on the mucous membranes of the bronchioles to reduce coughing. The action is mild and the taste pleasant, making it especially useful for children's colds or coughs. Traditionally, it has been used as an aid in whooping cough.

Red clover is known as an herbal alterative in that it acts gradually to change metabolism and tissue function to restore the body's balance. Accordingly, it is a useful adjunct in any acute or chronic illness. Its high mineral content (as a legume), combined with its alterative properties, make red clover a particularly useful support in eczema and psoriasis. It is thought that deficiency of certain trace minerals in the body sets the stage for conditions such as psoriasis or eczema to occur. The same trace minerals may also aid in digestion, another factor thought to be important in the chronic skin conditions. Red clover has also been used as supportive treatment in cancer with evidence to suggest that it inhibits tumor growth.

Red clover is simple to use and has no apparent toxicity. There are no contraindications to its use other than allergies to clovers in general or to red clover, specifically.

Harvesting: The flower heads can be gathered when the plant is in bloom. Blossoms that have begun to dry or fade should be avoided. The clover tops can be plucked from the top of the plant easily by hand. To dry for storage, spread flower heads out in a single layer on screens or cheesecloth to allow airflow all around them. Or dry them on brown bags, turning several times to permit even drying. Make sure clover is thoroughly dried before storing. Place in airtight containers when crumbly to the touch, and store out of the sun or other direct lighting.

Dosages: Pour 1 cup of boiling water over 1–2 teaspoons of dried clover blossoms, and let steep for 5 minutes. Cool to body temperature, and drink three to four times daily.

FROM THE AUTHOR'S JOURNAL
JUNE 16

This morning's trek out to the side field is hurried. Last night, mowing started, and I am afraid the chickweed will be gone before I get to gather more. Already a wide path has been carved around the field, dividing it into sections, so I'm out in a rush today to see what I can find. Long grass is matted in a row I walk along. Red clover and cinquefoil and yarrow are already wilting where they were cut. I start out at one edge of the field where the grasses look thinner, thinking it will be easier to find the tiny chickweed blossoms if the grass is sparse.

While I watch for chickweed, I start to pick red clover blossoms, and soon my bag fills with the purple flowers instead of chickweed. I meet some of my field neighbors, the spittlebugs. Lots of the clover stems have frothy places on them, and sometimes when I pluck a blossom whose bottom is covered with the foam, I get my fingers in it. I decide to sit down to work, thinking that at eye level with the plants, I can see underneath the blossoms to look for spittlebug drool.

Sitting low like this, I peer out across the field through purple clover heads and yellow cinquefoil, and the russet blossoms of sorrel, and a screen of green grasses. I feel like an animal, hidden and yet noticing everything.

Bugs join me. There is a whitish flying insect that must be a moth. Its fancy wings are thin and carved into a wedge shape. It likes the clover, too, and I wonder if it is drinking nectar. A stinkbug moves from one blossom to the next avoiding my fingers. There are no bees yet—it's too early in the day for them.

I glance up to check for another patch of clover to work at and gasp. The sun has slipped up while I was looking on the ground. It stands against a haze of gray, a perfect flame-colored circle wavering at the horizon. I can almost hear it move. Soon, my bag is full to bursting, and I head for home, trying not to see anymore clover because I could pick endlessly and would never get to work. Near the edge of the field, a patch of chickweed reclines against the grasses neighboring it, and I can't resist gathering a handful to add to my supply.

What wonderful work this herbing is. Sometimes I think I'm crazy for doing this work in a world that has no formal recognition of the subtler things. But this morning, in this field surrounded by purple clover heads, in peace and stillness under the flame-colored sun, I remember what matters to me, and am renewed.

Kitchen Notes

At home, I spread red clover blossoms out on a wide, round basket and set it between two windows in the herb room, where the new chick-weed lies on screens, added to yesterday's supply. The house smells like honey and freshness. Blue jays tap at seed on the dooryard porch, and I rush to get ready for work.

Experiences with Red Clover

Last winter I used red clover blossoms in a cough syrup where it added sweetness and color as well as healing. And only a few weeks ago, red clover went into a tea for a friend with mononucleosis. I used it, too, in early spring as a daily tea when the blackflies were bad and I had so many bites. It helped with the sick, droopy feeling I had after being bit-ten so many times. Now I use it every year during bug season.

COMFREY
Symphytum officinale

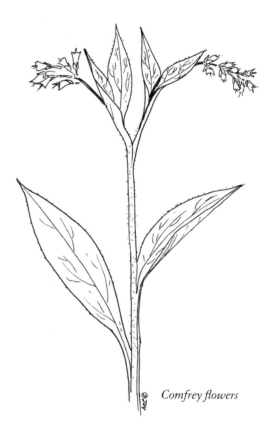

Reflections: Near the old pear trees where the deer come to eat, I dig a hole and plant a comfrey root and its bedraggled leaves. If this plant takes hold, deer can eat some in the spring and help to keep the comfrey under control. And when it spreads, I'll have my own supply nearby to watch over. The rain, falling harder now, slides through my hair and into my eyes, and I swipe at my face with a muddy hand. Hopefully, the rain will nurse this little root and give it a good start. I turn my face up to the sky in thanks, letting the rain wash away the mud, and then go back inside.

Comfrey flowers

Description: Comfrey is a tall, rough-leaved plant found growing in waste places and old fields. It can become a nuisance since it reproduces rapidly—even from just a tiny bit of root.

Comfrey roots grow deep in the soil and are covered with a dark brown bark that reveals a white inner core when cut. The stems and leaves are covered with coarse bristly hairs. Leaves are large near the bottom of the plant, up to 12 inches long, and get smaller toward the

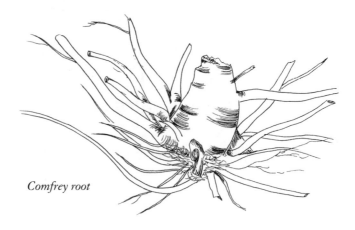

Comfrey root

top. The stalks of lower leaves are long, and when torn, they exhibit rubbery fibers that stretch before tearing. The leaves are lance or oval shaped, with softly pointed tips. They occur alternately along the stem and have simple, smooth margins. The leaves, stems, and roots all produce a very mucilaginous juice when cut or torn. Plant height is up to 3 or 4 feet.

Comfrey flowers are generally purplish blue, but may vary, ranging from white to pink with occasional yellowish tinges. The blossoms are bell shaped and occur in a raceme at the tip of curved stems throughout the summer. Flowers are ¹/₂ to 1 inch long, and die back to produce a cuplike capsule containing four seeds.

Medicinal Uses: Comfrey has several medicinal actions. It is known as a vulnerary and as an astringent. These properties make it useful in the healing of minor external wounds. Comfrey can be used for minor injuries of the skin, where it will work to increase cell production, causing wounds to heal over rapidly. Comfrey is also demulcent, producing a mucilage that coats and soothes irritated tissues. It will help reduce inflammation and at the same time lessen scarring. It has traditionally been used internally for stomach and duodenal ulcers for the same wound-healing effect, although this use is currently discouraged due to concern about certain toxic compounds in the plant.

Comfrey also has expectorant properties and has a relaxing effect on the respiratory membranes. Since it helps relax and soothe membranes, it has been traditionally used in coughs, asthma, and bronchitis.

Harvesting: Both leaves and root are used medicinally, with the root being a bit more potent and mucilaginous than the leaves. Leaves are gathered from the healthy plant any time during its growing season, although during flowering is the best time for a leaf harvest. Bundle the leaves in very small batches, and hang upside down out of the sun in a spot where there is good air circulation. Check the bundles daily to make sure that the leaves are not blackening or moldy.

Comfrey root can be dug in early spring, just as shoots emerge from the soil, or in the fall after frosts have killed off most of the leafy material. The roots should be dug, cleaned, and cut into thin slices. If roots are old and rough, the outer bark can be peeled off before drying. Store leaves and root when dried in airtight containers out of the sun.

Dosages: A tea or wash of comfrey leaves can be made by using 1 tablespoon of the dried leaves to 1 cup of boiling water. Pour water over leaves and let steep 15–20 minutes. A wash of the root is made by using 1 tablespoon of dried root in 1 cup of water, and simmering for 15–20 minutes. The strained decoction or infusion can used as a compress for wounds and skin irritations. Also, the dried leaves can be extracted into oil and the oil used as the base for an herbal salve for skin problems.

If used fresh, the bruised, fresh leaf is applied directly to the skin, and the cleaned, crushed root can be applied to a minor wound if desired. In minor burns, applying fresh comfrey leaf or root to the area can be helpful.

CAUTION: Potentially toxic pyrrolizidine alkaloids have been isolated in comfrey, and have been shown to be harmful to the liver if taken in large doses over long periods of time. Until further evidence clarifies the safety of internal use of comfrey, use should be limited to external application.

Finally it rains. Sometime in the night I heard it start and then heard nothing else. Now, at 5 AM, the sky has lightened a bit but is overcast and full of clouds, and a sprinkle continues. I know the garden is happy, and maybe this rain will help the brown and parched grasses in the field. Maybe it will rain all day. We sure could use it.

Today I am at a friend's house to gather comfrey from her field. Years ago a handful of comfrey seedlings were planted to use as feed for live-stock. The animals loved it but are long gone, and now comfrey has taken over close to half an acre. The plants that originally grew here have spread, and half the tillable land is packed with dark fuzzy leaves. My first year in Maine I lived here for a while and tried making a gar-den, but comfrey was a most invasive weed. I was constantly pulling up comfrey sprouts attached to fat, succulent roots. Since then, I've avoided planting it in my garden at home. Comfrey does grow wild, and wherever it is I'm sure there is lots of it. Since I haven't seen it in its natural state, I use this patch every year for my harvest—first for the leaves and then later in the fall for roots.

Now, I pile out of the car with my gear—garden snips and rubber bands and string, and a shovel just in case I decide to harvest a root. In the little field beside the barn, comfrey stands tall, packing the space with close, dark green leaves. Its purple flower curls are just beginning to unfold. Fat bumblebees buzz all around, and I have to be careful not to disturb them. They seem to love these blossoms. I finally settle into a rhythm of working. In the silence, I become aware of a noise that gets louder and louder, and I look up to see if there is a railroad track nearby, expecting a train. But the noise is only the field full of comfrey being worked by an army of bees.

I pull at the rough leaves one by one. Fibers in the leaf stems seem to stretch a little before they finally tear away. As I pull each leaf away from its stem, juice appears at the torn edge right away. When I put some to my tongue, it tastes green and fresh, a little slippery, and good. I can see why the animals liked it. Bundling the leaves together, I think how like cats' tongues they are, rough against my skin. Some of the larger leaves are almost painful to pick, they prickle so.

Once I have enough leaves for a winter's use, I decide to gather a few of the roots to have on hand, even though it's early in the season yet. So many plants are crowded together that when I dig one root, a knotted clump comes up. I cut into a fat root, and taste a slice. There is lots of mucusy juice at the cut end, and when I put a piece of the root on my tongue, it is slippery and at the same time strongly astringent—a funny combination. I heave the clump of knotted roots into my bag. There is surely enough to last until later in fall when I can harvest more. In the meantime, I gather up the bundles of comfrey leaves, the bag of roots, and other gear, and trek back to the car, heading for home.

Kitchen Notes

In the kitchen I spread some of the larger comfrey leaves out in a single layer along the bottom of a flat, shallow basket. The basket gets set between two windows where the air blows through constantly. Some of the leaves I hang in small bundles from the herb-drying rack, and these are the ones I'll keep my eye on. Last year my harvest of comfrey did not dry well. The bundles I made were large and thick, and the leaves in the middle of each batch blackened and rotted as the outer leaves dried. This year I'm being cautious, and will keep close watch on them. Only five or six leaves are gathered in each bundle, so they should do fine.

On the counter, a ball of roots waits to be cleaned. I rinse the roots under running water and scrub at them with a brush. One is as thick as my wrist, and the others are smaller. I slice the roots into thin bits so they will dry easily. They're beautiful, with a pure white inside and a blackish outer layer that is like hardened skin. And they're slippery. By the time I have sliced three roots, the first ones I cut are darkening already. Now, I'll spread them out, one layer deep, on a screen to dry.

I clean up soil and ragged plant scraps from the counter, and find one small root that I missed. It's a perfect size for planting, and I decide to risk putting it in the back field so I can have my own supply close to home. I throw plant scraps onto the compost pile and head out to the back field in another drizzle of rain.

Experiences with Comfrey

Every year comfrey is a main ingredient in a healing salve we use for wounds and scratches and sunburn. The dried leaves and roots go into olive oil along with other herbs for skin irritations—calendula and rose petals from the seaside, and chickweed if I have it on hand, and plantain. These get set aside to steep for a couple of weeks, and then the herbal oil that results gets poured off and heated with beeswax to make a salve. People at the local hospital where my sister works call it the "miracle salve" and ask for some routinely. They are constantly reporting on new things it helps to heal, so we keep making it up in large batches to share.

SWEET FERN
Comptonia peregrina

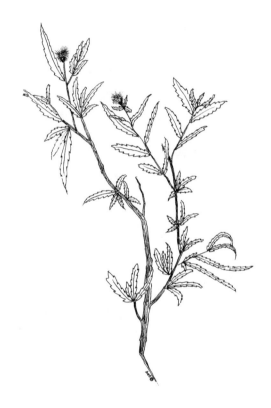

Reflections: Down by the development road, the cleared area where trees have been taken down is lush with bright new growth. The breeze blows wonderful scents at me—pine, dew-covered earth, and the strong, deep, heady smell of sweet fern. I find deer tracks and imagine that the animals must come here at night, after the construction crew has left and all is quiet, to stand like I do now, looking around at the changes. I imagine that they make new plans, or maybe they just wait, like I do, to see how much the development changes things. Maybe they can adapt. I worry for them, though.

Description: Sweet fern is a low-growing, deciduous shrub generally found in dry soil along roadsides and in fields along the edges of forest land. The plant is highly aromatic when crushed.

The leaves are alternate and occur along stiff, woody stems. The leaf margins are very wavy and fernlike, giving the plant its common name. Leaf length is up to 6 inches, and the leaves are dark green in color. They feel somewhat oily when crushed.

Sweet fern bears fruit in the form of a bristly, light green seed capsule that can be found on the plant in fall. Plant height is up to 5 feet.

Medicinal Uses: Externally, sweet fern has been used traditionally to relieve itching and irritation from such skin conditions as poison ivy, general rashes, insect bites, and shingles. The fresh leaves can also be crushed and rubbed on the skin to keep away insects for a short period of time. Internally, sweet fern acts as an astringent and is useful for mild diarrhea, stomach cramps, and indigestion. It is also useful as a mouthwash to help relieve gum inflammations and mouth sores.

Not much is known about sweet fern's actions since it has not been studied intensively. It has, however, had repeated uses in folkloric remedies in the Northeast.

Harvesting: Cut the leafy twigs from the plant any time during its growing season, spring through early fall. Remove individual leaves from the twigs, and dry by spreading out on screens or other appropriate material. Or the leafy twigs can be bundled to dry, and then the dried leaves stripped from them for storage.

Dosages: Externally, a strong tea of sweet fern leaves can be applied to the affected areas of skin on clean cloth several times a day. If a whole-body rash is evident, a bathtub can be filled with the strong tea, and the body soaked for 20 minutes several times a day.

Internally, an infusion can be made by using 1 rounded tablespoon of dried leaves to 1 cup of boiling water, and drunk several times a day.

FROM THE AUTHOR'S JOURNAL
JUNE 24

This morning is cold, just above 40 degrees, and the sumacs sway in a new wind. Birds feed noisily in the backyard, and sparrows and goldfinches vie for space at the birdbath. I am up a little later than usual, and by the time I pass the front windows, the rising sun is already painting fans of orange and coral across the sky. The windows of the barn and a neighbor's house glow like glass fragments in a kaleidoscope, holding bits of the sunrise as it changes.

As I walk, the brisk breeze and cooler temperatures have me huddled in a jacket with the hood pulled up—quite a treat after last week's almost 100 degrees! Down at Weeks's farm, the cows in the field are almost hidden in the tall grasses, and I imagine that they take some warm comfort from its protection. Only their flat brown backs show, gliding along as they feed.

Alongside the road, everything rustles in the breeze. Yarrow trembles in full bloom, and beside it the last of the buttercups shiver. Dogbane is full of pinkish flowers, and I remind myself to pick some for home on the way back. I walk along the development road, on straw spread by the logging crew to hold the soil in place, and make no sound.

In pockets in the tender growth of a clearing are some darker green splotches of sweet fern, rising bushy and lush. In early spring the woody stems were just sprouting lacy leaves, and even then the scent was wonderful. Now, sweet fern is in full growth, with the beginnings of its seed—pale, bristly heads—showing at the top of the stems.

I bend down to gather some now and strip off some of the leaves to crush and rub over my skin. A naturalist friend taught me that sweet fern will repel biting insects, so I try it now to discourage the blackflies that are bugging me. I wonder idly if I could use sweet fern in the woods to keep my human smell from scaring off the animals I like to watch. Native Americans sometimes used wild plants to rub on their bodies when they were hunting, to disguise their scent. I don't want to hunt, but I'd love to see more wildlife when I'm out.

As I stand there musing about covering my skin with sweet fern, holding my harvest, I hear a sharp huffing cough to the side of me, and a crashing sound, and just beside me, a white-tailed buck runs to leap away. As I watch, he gets smaller, and the woods close up behind him.

At the end of the road, where a house foundation stands, I walk around a bit, looking at the rough forest floor now bare of trees. Wintergreen stands bronzed by sun it hadn't seen before this year. I feel glad to have seen the deer, and sad to have invaded what little there is left of his territory here. These times are hard for the deer, I imagine. Two houses are going up here where a month ago there were only clearings. I never see moose tracks here anymore. Moose are too skittish to stick around when people start moving in.

Where will they all go, I wonder—the deer, the moose, and all the other animals? Do they wonder what's going on? How will they adapt? How will this invasion change their lives? Walking back up the road, I wish them well—I wish us all well—and take my sweet fern home.

Experiences with Sweet Fern

An herbalist friend told me that she used sweet fern on serious cases of poison ivy, making a strong tea of the dried leaves and then dipping a cloth in it to wrap around the rash. I've used it, too, in a bug bite balm I made up. It helped to soothe the insect bites, and I loved the heady scent it gave the salve. Sweet fern goes into an astringent powder I make with plantain and slippery elm. This powder gets mixed with water for a bug bite paste. It works so well I give it away to friends, and usually in the summer I am speckled with green when the blackflies are biting, or when I get stung by a bee.

PARTRIDGEBERRY
Mitchella repens

Reflections: This morning I move into the woods—over pine-needley earth and mossy rocks—and squat in a soft place. Canada mayflower is full of shiny greenish berries that are just forming. Under the low branches of pine, pyrola blooms. And at my feet, partridgeberry is in flower. Being in the woods like this soothes me. I watch the sun cut through the morning mist and the low clouds cluster and rise to disappear. A little breeze makes this day cooler than the last—all in all, another nice day!

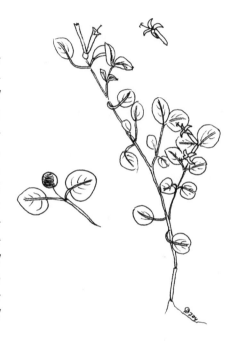

Description: An attractive evergreen woodland creeper with bright scarlet fruit, partridgeberry is a common forest ground cover in either damp or dryer woods. The plant is evergreen, and leaves may be found even under a snow cover.

The leaves are opposite, occurring in pairs along the stems. They are round in shape, $1/2$ to 1 inch long, and are dark, shiny green, often with white vein markings. The stems can grow up to 2 feet in length, creeping along the forest floor.

Partridgeberry flowers are small, $^1/_2$ inch in length. They are fragrant, white or pinkish tinged in color, and occur in pairs at the end of creeping stems. The blossoms have four petal-like lobes that erupt and curve outward from a long funnel-shaped corolla. The lobes are slightly hairy on the inside. Partridgeberry flowers in late spring and early summer.

The fruit is a bright red berry that forms from the twin flower at the end of creeping stems. The berries may be seen on the plant even into the following spring. They are edible, although mealy in texture and not very tasty.

Medicinal Uses: Partridgeberry is parturient, acting to prepare the reproductive system for labor and delivery. It was employed by the Native American women in the last few months of pregnancy to promote an easier birth. The herb is astringent, tonic to the reproductive system, and emmenagogue, and thus acts to tone and regulate the reproductive process. As an astringent and emmenagogue, the herb can be used to control excessive bleeding. The herb has also been used for men with chronic prostatitis, where it helps control symptoms.

Harvesting: Gather the aerial parts any time when it is actively growing, and especially during its season of bloom. Simply grasp the terminal end of a creeping stem and pull upward. The tiny rootlets that form along the stems will pull up easily, and the plant can be trimmed at its base. To dry, either bundle several stems together with a rubber band and hang to dry, or spread them loosely along a screen or basket material. When leaves or stems are brittle, they are ready to store. A fresh-plant tincture can also be made by placing the plant parts in alcohol soon after collection, and letting the mixture sit for 2 weeks. (Dried-plant tinctures can be made from stored plants at any time.)

HARVESTING CAUTION: Partridgeberry is another slow-growing, difficult to propagate woodland plant and is at risk in some states. Check with your local environmental association before harvesting.

Dosages: For tea, use 1 teaspoon of the dried plant to 1 cup of boiling water. Steep 10 minutes, and drink three times daily. If taking the tincture, either fresh- or dried-plant, use 30 drops ($^1/_4$ teaspoon) three times a day.

FROM THE AUTHOR'S JOURNAL
JUNE 27

This morning the mists are heavy in the field and hang like a low blanket just above the grass. Coming daylight lights them up. Everything is covered with dampness, and on the mountain, mist rises slowly, hanging like frosty breath in winter.

I go down to Big Sandy because it's been awhile since I was there and so much has grown up lately. Just down the hill, along the roadside, blackberry vines cover the soil. They are loaded with blossoms, and I remind myself to come here to pick in a month or so. Sapling trees are overgrown and lean into the road, and I try to find the willows I worked on, but can't.

I take a path to the clearing and look at the ground and at leaves glittery with raindrops for so long that everything blends and shimmers. What light there is gleams on every damp leaf, silver. At the path's edge, partridgeberry spreads out over rusty pine needles; it is in full bloom. The flowers that tip the viny plant now are fragrant and pinkish-white. Each plant bears twin flowers, a lovely glistening pair, whose petals seem to have fuzzy hairs on top of them.

All early spring I waited for partridgeberry to bloom and finally gave up, thinking I had missed its flowering season. The leaves are always easy to recognize—roundish dark green pairs of leaves, divided by white midveins. They cover the forest floor from the earliest spring right through the snows and are probably there even through winter, just covered up.

Now, I'm so happy to see this herb in bloom, I start gathering it right away. I pick up the flowering tip, grasp the stem, and pull upward. Some ends snap off after a few inches, and some come up long. When I pull up one strand, others come with it. They are bound together along a web of connecting roots like a woven mat. Some strands pull up a path through the pine needle litter and before I put them in the bag, I pick out humusy debris and pine needles, and pinch off whatever leaves are yellowed.

I pick a few lengths that still bear last year's berries, plump and brilliant red. Everywhere I look, there is more partridgeberry, and soon my bag is full of it, scarlet berries showing bright and clear.

On the way back home, I pick a few still-healthy sprigs of self-heal, an armful of sweet fern to dry, and one tiny plant with an odd-shaped flower called cow wheat. I smile to myself, thinking how I must look— arms full of plants, a bag of special partridgeberry dangling from one hand, and a dainty specimen to press held carefully in the other. Back up the hill, I turn to look behind me. The sun has hit the blue ridges of the mountain. A breeze starts and rustles through the plants I hold, and through my hair.

Experiences with Partridgeberry

Last year I made a tincture of the fresh partridgeberry plants, but my supply is gone now. I love offering it to women for menstrual irregularities. I give it, too, in the last few months of pregnancy, to tone and strengthen the uterus. Last year I gave some to a friend who was having trouble with cramping and irregular menstrual cycles, mostly as a tonic and regulator, and it helped. I put partridgeberry in formulas, too, for women discontinuing the birth control pill, and it helped them regain a normal cycle. I've used it along with other herbs to help in menopause, and have found it dependable. I've also used partridgeberry in formulas for men with prostatitis, and it works—a truly nondiscriminating herb!

MULLEIN
Verbascum thapsis

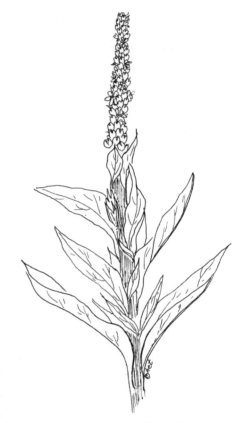

Reflections: I'm out earlier than usual this morning—4:45 AM—to try to beat the bugs. I take a well-worn path, and at its bend, along a dry ditch, the mullein I've come for is tall and flowering. A smokey blue haze keeps all its colors mute this early, and the sunny yellow blossoms are just brighter shades of gray.

Description: Mullein is common along roadsides and in waste places and is not very particular about growing conditions. It can stand up to 8 feet tall and can be recognized easily even in winter, when dried and darkened stem and flower spikes stand tall above snowy fields. It is generally a biennial, with a two-year life cycle.

Mullein leaves are a primary identification feature in this plant. They are large, up to 1¹/₂ feet in length and half as wide, and are oblong or oval in shape. The leaves are alternate and covered with soft downy hairs that give the leaves and stem a velvety feel. Leaves generally have smooth margins, although in some plants there is slight toothing. In its first year, the plant appears as a basal rosette of fuzzy leaves, and in its second year, it sends up a thick central stalk bearing leaves that get progressively smaller. The stalk is topped with a fat flower spike.

The flowers are bright yellow, with five petals. They occur along the thick flower spike at the top of the tall stem. The flowers themselves are stalkless. The blossoms are up to 1 inch wide. Mullein blooms early summer through fall.

Medicinal Uses: All parts of the mullein plant can be used. The leaves and blossoms are expectorant, demulcent, and sedative. Mullein has long been used as a general tonic and remedy for any problems of the respiratory tract. The leaves can be taken on a regular basis as an aid for chronic asthma or bronchitis, where they have a tonic effect. The flowers and leaves not only act to reduce inflamed mucous membranes, but also act as a mild respiratory sedative.

Mullein is appropriate for treating colds where there is mild chest congestion since it helps soften mucus, making it easier to cough up.

The blossoms of mullein used in an oil base are helpful for treating earaches. Mullein root is mildly diuretic and astringent, and it can be used to aid in preventing bed-wetting or loss of bladder control.

Harvesting: The leaves can be gathered any time during growing season. Cut leaves from the plant near their base, and clean thoroughly since the hairs often attract insects or hold bits of roadside fluff. Spread leaves out on screens or baskets to dry, turning occasionally. Since the leaves are so fleshy, they may take up to 2 weeks to dry.

Dosages: Use 1–2 tablespoons of dried leaves to a cup of boiling water. Let steep 15–30 minutes, and drink three times a day. If using an oil of the blossoms for earaches, warm oil gently and place 1–2 drops in the affected ear several times daily.

This morning I walk along the Porter Road, hoping to make the 3-mile circle back to the house. The last few times I tried it, the mosquitoes were bad and I had to turn back, swatting and flapping at my head until I reached home. Today is better. It's a chilling morning, around 50 degrees, and a breeze blows. Down at Weeks's farm, the cows are still lounging on the hay when I pass, and Boomer, the dog, won't be making his compost rounds until 5:30 or so when the farmer gets up to milk.

Up the hill there are two dead chipmunks in the road that weren't there yesterday. They lie within 10 feet of each other, and I stop to look, wondering what happened. Were they crossing the road together, or did one get killed first and the other come to investigate? There are so many roadkills lately. It makes me sad to find them, but I do get to see animals up close that I wouldn't see otherwise. The real consolation, though, is knowing there is a variety of wildlife nearby. It makes me feel that despite life's occasional cruelty and hectic pace, there is still a vital balance maintained in this area.

I reach the road I wanted, and see Solomon's seal forming berries already. The leaves are yellowing and drying at the edges. I want to keep track of these plants until the fall, when I can gather roots. If I watch every week, maybe it will be easier to find them again. Along the roadside, greenery is lush with baby trees—oak, maple, some pine, a few beech, and the wild cherries. Wild sarsaparilla and ferns have taken over, and the smaller stuff is being crowded out or overgrown. The patch of trillium I saw in early spring is dying back. Lots of meadow rue pokes up, 6 feet tall or more. Now that I've found it in one place, I see it everywhere—in groups of two or three plants—with fluffy white flowers and beautiful leaves. It's on my list of herbs to gather soon.

Next to it, at a bend in the path, is the mullein I've come for today. It's one of my favorite plants—so abundant, so ignored, and with so many uses! Already this season I have gathered some of its leaves to use for tea. Now that the flowers are out, I decide to gather some to use for an earache oil. The blossoms are a wonderful, sunny yellow, the brightest color in this pale, early day. I gather them, one by one, and place them in a bag. Insects must like this plant as much as I do, for all along the flower spike, small, shiny black bugs move. I shake one out of a blossom before putting is in the bag. I decide to pick more fuzzy leaves, too, and pick around a daddy longlegs hiding in the close niches where leaves join the stem.

On the way home, I see a little dead garter snake at the edge of the dirt road. He has a tiny bloody hole poked in one side, but otherwise is perfect. I turn him over and he feels supple in my fingers. His ribs move like dominos would fall—one following the other in a fluid motion. His belly is a rusty-color red. I wonder what killed him—some large bird, maybe. Near the end of the road, the usual dogs come out to bark at me, and I yell at them or talk, depending on their mood.

Kitchen Notes

At home, today's leaves go to the screen to dry, next to the last harvest of mullein. The bright flowers go into a little jar and get covered with olive oil. They sit now on the windowsill in the sun where they will stay for a couple of weeks. Then I'll strain out the old blossoms and bottle the oil to use, one drop at a time. Before the snows come, I'll probably gather more leaves and blossoms to get us through the winter—and to share, too, if need be.

Experiences with Mullein

Mullein was one of the first herbs I used, mostly for a daughter's asthma. The leaves went into a daily tea along with coltsfoot and comfrey. Now she doesn't need it every day. When the pollen count is high, or when she has the beginnings of a cold, mullein is still what she turns to for support, and she's been able to stay off medication with its help.

RASPBERRY
Rubus idaeus and species

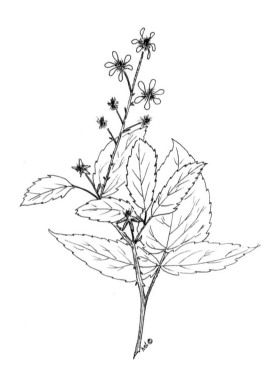

Reflections: It is 5 AM, and I'm hoping to foil the bugs and get out and home before the heat starts up again. Along the last bend in the road, where the surface is still soil rather than asphalt, raspberry grows right up to he cleared roadway and is tall and full of fruit. I eat a few fat berries as I pick, and work quietly. Bullfrogs twang, and the birds I disturbed start up again. Maybe if I am silent and still, and just work at gathering, they will think I am one of them.

Description: Raspberry is a prickly stemmed, spreading plant bearing edible fruit and is common to roadsides, thickets, and disturbed areas. Several species are indigenous throughout the United States. The wild red raspberry, *Rubus idaeus,* is common to roadsides and clearings in many areas, and is the official raspberry of herbal tradition.

Raspberry leaves are alternate and divided, with three to five sharply and irregularly toothed leaflets. They are bright green, often with whitish undersides, and occur along a stiff, erect, prickly stem. The stems are often arched and form dense thorny thickets. Plants may grow up to 6 or 7 feet in height.

The flowers are white or cream colored, with five regular petals. The petals and sepals are roughly the same length. Blossoms, about 1/2 inch wide, appear in late spring and early summer.

The fruit is a soft, juicy, multisegmented berry that is edible and ripens in mid- to late summer. The berries are juicy and sweet, with fleshy fruit surrounding many seeds. They are used for making wild jams, jellies, and syrups.

Medicinal Uses: Raspberry leaves are astringent and tonic, and they have a special function for the tissues of the female reproductive system. A tea of raspberry leaves helps tone the muscles of the uterus and has been used for centuries to help prepare the system for childbirth. Its astringency makes it useful during and after birth, where it will help control bleeding. Raspberry tea can also be used to help reduce heavy menstrual bleeding and, in general, to tone and normalize the reproductive system's functions. It is helpful to use after miscarriages or abortion to help restabilize the system.

Raspberry leaves and root bark can be used, too, to help control diarrhea, since its astringency tones inflamed or irritated tissues. In this case, other species of raspberry can be used interchangeably, as all share the same properties of astringency.

Harvesting: It is best to wear thick, protective gloves when gathering raspberry. Cut leaves from the stems any time when the plant is in full growth, and especially when it is flowering. Handle carefully, and spread to dry on screens, baskets, or paper bags.

To use the root bark, dig up medium-sized plants after leafy material has died back in the fall. Wash roots carefully, and strip off outer bark. Spread out to dry on screens or baskets, and store when dry. Bark strips can be cut into small pieces for tea, or then powdered in a blender and mixed with honey to treat diarrhea.

Dosages: Raspberry is water soluble and works fine as an infusion. Use 1 tablespoon of chopped dried leaves to 1 cup of boiling water, steep 15–30 minutes, and drink two or three times daily. A tincture, made from the fresh or dried leaves, can be added to other herbs for the female reproductive system. To use the root bark for diarrhea, simmer 1 tablespoon of root in $1^{1}/_{2}$ cups of water for 10 minutes. Strain and drink every 2 hours.

FROM THE AUTHOR'S JOURNAL
JULY 8

This morning is another hot one. In the east, haze makes the sky look mean, and the sun coming up burns through shadows. Today I walk down the development road near the porcupine house because last time I was there the raspberry leaves were tender and green. It looked like a good place to harvest them. Down the sloping road, I crunch on gravel and keep an eye out for deer—or bear—until I come to the spot where raspberry grows right up to the cleared path. Its thorny runners snake along the ground, holding soil in place that used to be forest floor.

Early in the spring, these bushes were covered with white blossoms where now berries hang. A few of the plants still have flowers, but most are full of ripe or green fruit. I pick a place to start and work with scissors and garden gloves. The raspberry bushes are covered with sharp thorns that line even the veins underneath the leaves. I hold onto each leaf tip, cut at the base of the leaf cluster, and gingerly place each group of leaves in the bag. The perfect, tender green leaves are the ones I gather. The older, darker leaves might have different properties. Maybe someday I'll harvest two different batches, young leaves and old, and compare notes on the different effects. For now, the tenderest leaves go into the bag. Any that look bedraggled or bug-bitten get left behind.

I eat while I work. The raspberries are sweet and just melt away to nothing in my mouth. Working quietly, I keep an eye out for the bear I saw running into the nearby woods last week. Not that I mind sharing berries, but I'm afraid the bear might!

The bag fills with bright raspberry leaves, and my belly fills with fruit. The sweet scent of berries lifts from the bushes where I work.

Near the little streambed that is dry now, I step into a cluster of brambles and pick a few berries, then walk farther down the path to pick again. Suddenly, the bushes rustle loudly, and shake a bit, and I realize I have surprised some small animal. I talk to it, apologizing to whatever it is, hoping I've not intruded on a skunk. The bushes quiver again, then quiet down. I pick for a while longer, then leave for home.

Kitchen Notes

At home, there are so many raspberry leaves I can't find drying space for all of them. They spread out like a hand and take up more space than I counted on. The basket fills with a layer of raspberry leaves, and then the screens fill. What is left over I decide to tincture, and chop into small bits with the scissors. These go into a jar and get covered with alcohol. It will be nice to have tincture to use in formulas.

Five days later, the leaves have shriveled up to one-third their original size. Although they feel dry, they don't quite crumble when I crush them, so they'll have to wait a few more days to be stored. The tincture is dark green now, almost opaque. It will sit for another week or so before I bottle it. I sip a cup of raspberry leaf tea now, remembering how much I like its fruity taste and scent. Noticing how much the leaves have shrunk in size, I decide I'll need to harvest more. The leaves should be fine to pick right up through fall. If I go soon, I can snack on raspberries again while I work.

Experiences with Raspberry

I've used raspberry leaves for all kinds of female reproductive system problems, and I use it, too, just for toning the tissues. A friend recently told me that his wife used raspberry leaf tea to help control bleeding during and after delivery of their home-birthed child, and that it did a fine job. Such a delightful use for this joyful herb!

SUNDEW
Drosera species

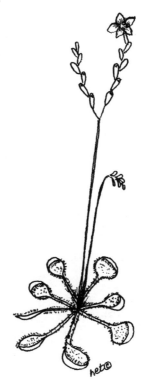

Reflections: Visiting a tiny island off the coast of Maine, I walk into a gravel pit that is covered with wildflowers. The place was once used as a source of sand to spread on the island's winter-frozen roads. The pit is abandoned now, and tucked into one craggy corner is tiny sundew, sparkling in the sun. I pick a few of the plants, shaking sand from their shallow roots and picking out a few ants. Crimson, dewy drops cling to my fingers, and I lick them off.

Description: Sundews are small insectivorous plants found growing in boggy areas or in wet, sandy, sterile soil. The whole plants are small—generally between 4 and 12 inches in width—and occur in colonies.

Several species of sundew occur in New England, and all may be used interchangeably. Local field guides are useful for species identification by the leaves, which vary in shape from round to thread-leaved.

In all sundews, the leaves are covered with reddish hairs, and the hairs have glands that exude dewlike drops of a sticky substance that traps insects. All species have shallow root systems.

Sundew flowers occur in one-sided racemes and vary in color from white to lavender. Blossoms have five petals and are $^1/_4$ to $^1/_2$ inch wide. Flowers occur June through September.

Medicinal Uses: Sundew is antispasmodic, demulcent, and expectorant. The whole plant can be used in tea or tincture form to aid in relieving respiratory infections. Sundew will promote the expectoration of mucus and help soothe irritated membranes and lessen cough. It can also help ease the coughs of asthma, bronchitis, and whooping cough, as well as other spasmodic coughs. Sundew has been proven to act against staph, strep, and pneumonia bacteria.

Harvesting: The whole plant, root and all, can be gathered any time during its growing season, although it is preferable to pick when flowering if possible. Rinse soil from roots, and wash any debris from the plants under gentle running water. Dry the plant by spreading on screens, cheesecloth, or brown paper bags, and turn every few days until brittle. Store the dried plant in airtight containers out of the sun. Dried- or fresh-plant tincture can be made by immersing the plant in alcohol, and setting aside in a darkened place for two weeks.

HARVESTING CAUTION: Some species of sundew are at risk. Be certain to check with your local environmental association for plant status before harvesting.

Dosages: To use sundew tincture, take 15–30 drops three or four times daily. For tea, use 1 tablespoon of dried, chopped plant to 1 cup of boiling water, steep 10 minutes, and drink three to four times daily.

CAUTION: No obvious toxicity has been reported, but it is best to start with small dosages. There are no apparent contraindications.

It's another searing day full of heat—85 degrees at 7 AM and 90 degrees by 9. We breathe slowly, and move slowly—and then only if we have to. Breezes are worshipped, and we move chairs into any window draft, even if it puts us in the middle of a room in an awkward spot. We argue about infinitesimal things. At the lake where we usually go to cool off, the water is tepid and not much help.

Today I may get some relief. From Portland, I'll take the ferry out to Long Island to do an herb walk and see what plants are growing there now. The ocean should at least have a breeze.

The drive to the ferry in Portland is hot, awful, and I get a headache from the glaring sun. On the boat, though, things get better. The ocean is green and clear, and the air smells salty and wet. A breeze blows foam over us and feels terrific. We cross the wake from other boats and bob side to side. By the time we reach the island, I am better. The air temperature is at least 10 degrees cooler than it was inland.

I visit with a friend for a while, and talk herbs and islands and development. We watch cardinals with their babies at the bird feeder. We walk, then, the island's perimeter—along the sandy roads, through woods, and down to the beach. We identify plants; wild roses grow like a fencing hedge all along the shore. At the roadsides, fireweed is just opening and so is yarrow. Blueberry bushes are full of fruit, and the blackberries are flowering. Along a path that ridges the shore the wild cherry trees grow; their bark can be gathered later in the season for coughs. The horsetail along the beach is much taller than it is inland. Dulse and Irish moss lie along the beach, and I pick some up for home.

We walk through an abandoned gravel pit now overgrown with wildflowers. In an area of the pit that stands in water early in the spring, we discover a real treat. Sundew, a relative of Venus's flytrap, stands crowded in the dry and gravelly soil. Its roundish leaves are full of tiny hairs covered with a bright red, gel-like liquid. When I touch a leaf, it leaves a stickiness on my finger. In my mouth, the gel has no taste. I chew up a leaf, and it gets slippery after a few bites.

The plants are exotic and beautiful, and are just beginning to flower. I haven't used sundew yet, because up to now I've not found it. I expected them to inhabit boggy earth, but the plant books say that any nutrient-poor and sandy soil will do. I'd like to take some home to try to transplant, but I'm afraid they'd wilt and die during the trip. I decide to gather some for tincture, and carefully pull up a few whole plants. Flower stalks full of buds protrude from the center of the basal leaves. Sticky red juice clings to my fingers as I pick, and I lick it off. I place each tender plant into the bag, lick my fingers again, and get ready to catch the ferry back to Portland. At the dock the air has cooled even more, and I am chilly as I wait for the boat. Cormorants feed in the shallow water as we sail off.

Back in Portland the air is hot again, and at home heat still hangs smugly at the 100 degree mark, making the house like an oven. At least I have memories of the island trip, and a bag of sundew to prepare.

Kitchen Notes

I get ready to tincture the sundew, cleaning the roots free of soil and breaking the plant into small bits. Grain alcohol gets poured over the pieces. The liquid turns orangey, and I sit watching it, licking my fingers clean. By bedtime, the little jar of sundew is dark orange. I poke a finger in the liquid and taste alcohol and slight sweetness. In a couple of weeks it will be ready to use. A pelting rain now cools the air, and I finally sleep, dreaming of ocean islands and sundew.

SHEPHERD'S PURSE
Capsella bursa-pastoris

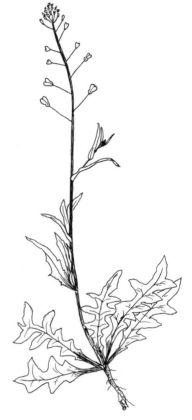

Reflections: It hasn't really rained here for weeks, and this morning I notice how brown and dry the grass is. Only in one place along the edge of the garden near the field is there a lush-looking patch of green. When I get close enough, I find shepherd's purse in bloom and bearing heart-shaped seedpods. Such a pretty little plant, its delicate looks belie its strength. I decide to start gathering this year's supply, and sit in the cool grass to work.

Description: A Mustard family member, shepherd's purse is a common weed and a fairly hardy plant found in gardens, lawns, roadsides, ditches, and waste places. It thrives where water is available, but it will grow in dry, rubbly soil as well. It is often eaten as one of the first spring greens and has a mild peppery taste like many members of the Mustard family.

The leaves occur at the base of the plant and along the thin stem. Basal leaves are irregularly divided or lobed and may be up to 4 inches long. Stem leaves are smaller and sparse, arrow shaped, and have bases that clasp the stem. The plant may attain 18 inches in height.

The flowers of shepherd's purse are very tiny, up to only $1/12$ inch in width. They are white and grow in a cluster atop the central stem. There are four even petals. Shepherd's purse blooms throughout its growing season—very early spring through late fall and even into winter.

The fruit makes the plant easy to identify. It occurs along the top third of the central stem in the form of a small triangular pod with an indentation at the tip, giving it the appearance of a small green heart. The seedpod was thought to be shaped like a shepherd's purse, hence its common name.

Medicinal Uses: Shepherd's purse is astringent, diuretic, and a mild uterine stimulant. It can be used to help stop excessive menstrual bleeding by regulating the cycle gently. As an astringent and uterine stimulant, it helps to normalize function while gently reducing menstrual flow. Because shepherd's purse is a uterine stimulant, it should not be used during pregnancy. However, it is helpful during labor and especially just after birth, where it will help tone the uterine tissues and control bleeding.

As an astringent, shepherd's purse can also be used in mild diarrhea, especially if bleeding is involved. Externally, the fresh plant can be crushed and applied to fresh wounds once they have been cleaned, where it will help stop slow bleeding and reduce inflammation.

Because of its diuretic action, shepherd's purse can be used in any kind of fluid retention, where it will act to promote the flow of urine. This action, combined with its astringency, makes it a helpful herb in the premenstrual symptoms of bloating with water retention and cyclic irregularity. In this case, it can aid in reducing edema and may help regulate the cycle.

Harvesting: Gather the whole plant any time during its growing season, and especially when it is in flower. Be sure that the plant is fresh when you gather it. (Often some of the plant leaves will appear green even while seedpods are dry and fading, and therefore the plant is not of much use.) Bundle the plants at the bases, and hang to dry. Once the plant parts feel crumbly, cut and store. A fresh-plant tincture can be made to add to other herbs for the female reproductive system. If desired, make the fresh-plant tincture soon after gathering the herb, and use it in place of the fresh or dried herb.

Dosages: For an infusion, use 1–2 tablespoons of dried plant material to 1 cup of boiling water. Let steep for 20 minutes. If using for menstrual bleeding or as an aid after birth, use 1 cup of tea every 1–2 hours until bleeding comes under control. For other problems, use 1 cup of tea three times daily. If using the tincture, use $1/4$ to $1/2$ teaspoonful three times daily for most conditions, and every 2 hours for help after birth.

FROM THE AUTHOR'S JOURNAL
JULY 13

Outside at 5 AM, I decide to go down to the back woods to see if the lobelia is up. I usually find it there in early summer, and the last time I was down, small plants with look-alike leaves had sprouted along the path. That was weeks ago, so today I can look for the flowers.

Out across the field, I worry about getting my shoes wet, but there is little moisture. The grasses in the back field look dry and golden tan, like a ripe grain harvest. All the red clover is topped with blackened flower heads. Cinquefoil has seeded already. A few yarrows are still flowering, but the grasses are browning and have brittle edges. Nothing looks lush anymore. The blueberry bushes are loaded with green fruits. Hopefully, we'll get some rain soon so the berries can come in juicy.

In the woods, bugs attack me—mosquitoes and deerflies. They buzz around my head and land on exposed skin. I resort to a head net finally, and the bugs hover nearby. This year they have been worse than usual. I always thought they liked moisture, but maybe it is heat that brings them out. Or maybe they are after the moisture and minerals on my skin. They make me walk faster than I normally would, and I look for lobelia quickly. No flowers have appeared yet, so I race back through the woods, swatting at the bugs who bite me through my shirt and through the netting. Near the garden at home, I spot shepherd's purse, growing lush and green despite the dry weather, and sit to gather some. I'm not surprised to find it in the lawn. Shepherd's purse is a tough and tenacious little plant, despite its daintiness. It sprouts in the vegetable garden along with other weeds, and springs up tall in the grass whenever we don't mow. I've even seen shepherd's purse popping up through cracks in the city sidewalks, heedless of its surroundings.

Now, I pull at a plant and it comes up root and all. Tiny white flowers are open at the top, and beneath are seedpods that stand out along the stem. At the base, leaves are ruffly and divided, and spread out in a flat circle. I just pick for a while. Being still, sitting on the lawn in the cool grass, quiet, picking one green thing and then another, settles me. I want to sit forever doing this.

I pop a piece in my mouth. This is the heaviest day of my period so later, at work, I'll drink shepherd's purse tea to regulate the flow. Now, sitting in the grass, I take my medicine simple. It tastes fine, not peppery like some mustards would. The piece in my mouth is fibrous, and I spit it out after a while, but like the flavor it leaves.

Kitchen Notes

Inside the kitchen, I clean the shepherd's purse, cut it up and put it into alcohol. Last year I gathered enough of this herb to use through several seasons. A quart jar of the dried plant still sets in the herb cupboard. But I've used up the tincture, taking it places where I couldn't make tea easily. Now, I'll replenish my supply. The alcohol is bright, light green already, and darkening by the minute. Shepherd's purse is one of my favorite herbs—simple to pick, simple to find, and simple to use. I chew another sprig, and get ready for work.

PIPSISSEWA
Chimaphila umbellata and *maculata*

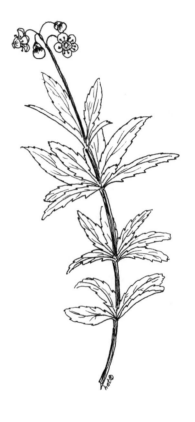

Reflections: Today is a perfect Maine summer day. The thermometer on the barn says 68 degrees. The morning air is clear and dry, and the sky is brilliant blue. The woods smell fresh and sweet. Next to the lush wintergreen, full of fat nodding buds, I find pipsissewa in bloom at last, her flowers as perfect as this day.

Description: Pipsissewa is a small, pretty evergreen plant of dry woods. Two *Chimaphila* species grow in the Northeast, and they can be used interchangeably as they have the same medicinal properties. Both species grow in dry woods, usually near pines or other conifers, and are found in colonies.

The official pipsissewa, *Chimaphila umbellata,* has leaves that are dark green and shiny. The plant is evergreen and can be found looking fresh even under snow cover. The leaves are stemless, finely toothed, and are lance shaped, widening at the tops. The leaves occur in whorls and can grow up to 3 inches in length. Plant height is generally between 3 and 10 inches.

Pipsissewa has pretty blossoms with five regular petals that are somewhat concave and reflexed. The flower is white, or pinkish white, and the petals surround a knobby green pistil. Surrounding the pistil are ten dark maroon-colored stamens. The blossoms are $^1/_3$ to $^1/_2$ inch across and occur in nodding clusters atop a central stem. The plant blooms in summer, June through August. After flowering, the plant produces brown seed capsules that remain on the dried stem throughout the winter and can be found on some plants the next spring.

Chimaphila maculata, another *Chimaphila* species, is commonly known as spotted or striped wintergreen. Flowers are very similar to those of pipsissewa, but the plant is just a bit shorter, up to 9 inches, and the leaves are more sharply pointed. The leaves can occur in whorls or along the stem and are mottled with whitish markings along the veins.

Medicinal Uses: Pipsissewa is diuretic, disinfectant, and antiseptic, and it is used to help relieve problems of the urinary tract. It can be used to treat mild urinary tract infections and the tendency to form kidney stones. Pipsissewa is especially helpful where there is a strong demand to urinate, but little urine is produced and it is cloudy. Pipsissewa is helpful, too, in chronic urinary tract infections where symptoms of urgency and burning are prominent. A tea of the herb can also be helpful in chronic prostatitis. Pipsissewa is sedative to the urinary tract and can be helpful with pain from this condition or from any of the urinary tract disorders. It can be used on a long-term basis for chronic kidney weakness.

Pipsissewa has another use. It can be taken at the beginning of a measles or chicken pox infection, where it will help to bring out the spots, making the duration of the disease shorter, and the patient more comfortable.

Harvesting: Gather the aerial parts as the herb is coming into flower. Harvest carefully, and avoid disturbing roots. Pipsissewa, like many woodland plants, propagates slowly, and it is best to gather only $^1/_4$ to $^1/_3$ of any population. The stems on this plant are fairly short and may be hard to bundle. If enough stem material is available, bundle and hang to dry. Otherwise, simply spread the plant material out on screens or baskets, and dry out of the sun. Store when leaves crumble easily. A fresh-plant tincture may be made upon gathering.

HARVESTING CAUTION: Although pipsissewa is an excellent urinary tract tonic and support and has no known toxicity, it is a slow-growing woodland plant that is difficult to propagate. Most states recommend that the plant not be harvested commercially or in sizeable amounts for personal use. Check with your local environmental agencies for status of this plant before harvesting.

Dosages: To use as a tea, place 1 tablespoon of chopped dried leaves into 1 1/2 cups of water, and simmer 15–20 minutes. Drink three times daily. If using the tincture, take 15–30 drops three times daily. For chronic kidney weakness or prostatitis, a cup of tea taken daily should suffice as a preventive and urinary tract tonic.

FROM THE AUTHOR'S JOURNAL
JULY 14

At 7:30 AM, the sun comes up and lights everything golden. A little breeze rustles the sumacs in the back and the elderberry leaves. Poppies flutter and bees hover just above each flower, waiting for the wind to die so they can dive again for nectar. A blue jay feeds at the dooryard steps. Sweet peas are bright and tall against the side of the house. Today is fine—bright and clear and sunny with blue skies. The air feels terrific.

This morning I will gather pipsissewa. All spring and during part of summer we've had so far, I've kept an eye on this plant. Today, I drive across town to the lake, to a woods of pine and hemlock and fir and a few hardwoods. Bushy shrubs line the edges of the forest, and sun glints on the lake as I make my way to the pipsissewa.

I often find this plant as soon as the snow melts in spring, because it is evergreen. And because I see it so early, I think it should flower right away, but it takes its time. Weeks ago these plants had buds—graceful, curvy-necked buds with bent and blushing heads held tight on a single stem. Now the flowers have opened, and they're amazing. Each one has five pale, pinkish white petals that are roundish and curved, flaring back from the center. The stamens are paired, dark maroonish brown, and stand around the central disk. The center is green, bulbous, with a flattened disk that is sticky with a vaguely sweet-tasting substance. Such an intricate and beautiful flower, it was certainly worth waiting for.

I pick pipsissewa now, breaking the plant off above the bottom group of leaves so I don't disturb its roots. Like other woodland plants, pipsissewa is a slow grower and difficult to cultivate, so I am careful to gather only a small portion of what stands here. I chew on a leathery leaf, and my mouth puckers with its astringency. My bag is soon half-filled, and this little population of plants can't stand to lose many more members. I bid the plants good-bye, and thank them, then leave the woods for midmorning sun. As the weeks pass, I can come back to watch pipsissewa make the transition to seedpod, watch them until the snows come, and then in the spring, start my vigil all over again.

Kitchen Notes

At home, I take my harvest out to process it. Some of the pretty petals have fallen off and lie on the dark tabletop like tiny porcelain cups. I scoop them up and cut them into pieces along with the whole plants, then put them in a jar with alcohol. It seems a shame to chop up all the plants though, so I save out one to put in the plant press. I arrange its leaves and blossoms and it looks perfect. The jar full of tincture makings goes into the herb cabinet, and the table gets cleaned of pretty scraps.

Experiences with Pipsissewa

Pipsissewa was one of the first herbs I gathered and used, and every year I collect a small supply. I use it alone, or put it in formulas with other urinary tract herbs. A few weeks ago, it went in small doses to a woman who had recurrent urinary tract problems, not so much to treat a current infection as to help tone and support the tissues of that system, and to act as a preventive. I've also used pipsissewa for interstitial cell cystitis, a potentially autoimmune affliction of the bladder, and it has helped to relieve the symptoms.

BLUEBERRY
Vaccinium species

Reflections: This morning I follow a darkened path in the dew-silvered grass where a doe has crossed the field, and come to the blueberry bushes full of ripening fruit. I pick and eat for a while, thinking how like the deer I am. We are glad for this day, content to be feeding easily, happy for the wind that blows bugs away, happy for the cooler time, happy for sun that warms our skin and ripens what we eat.

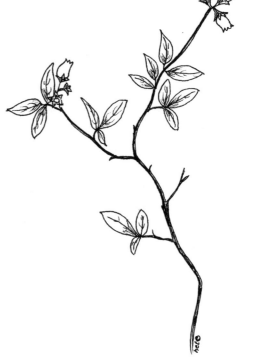

Description: Blueberry is a deciduous, woody shrub with alternate or clustered leaves and edible fruit. A number of varieties grow in the northeastern states. Check a field guide for specific identification in your area. Two common species in our region are the highbush blueberry and the lowbush blueberry.

Highbush blueberry, *Vaccinium corymbosum,* has leaves that are $1^1/2$ to 3 inches long and are smooth and elliptical in shape. They are slightly hairy underneath. The plant's height ranges from 3 to 15 feet. The white or whitish pink flowers are $1/4$ to $1/2$ inch long. The flowers occur in clusters at the ends of branches. Fruit is a dark dusky blue, round, and edible berry with deep flavor and sweet taste. The highbush blueberry grows in woods, swamps, or pastures. Flowers occur in spring and early summer, and fruit is ripe June through August, although some ripe fruit may remain on the branches later if not eaten by birds and animals.

Lowbush blueberry, *Vaccinium angustifolium,* is most often found in dry open soil. Leaves are finely toothed, $1/2$ inch wide, and about 1 inch in length. Flowers are white or pinkish white, and occur in clusters. Flowers bloom in spring and early summer. The fruit is a dark blue, edible berry that is sweet tasting. Fruit ripens May through August and, again, may remain on branches until later.

Medicinal Uses: A tea of blueberry leaves is astringent and diuretic and can be used to treat urinary tract infections where it will have an antiseptic effect. Blueberry leaves also help inhibit uric acid formation, making it useful in gout. Blueberry's leaves are often used, along with those of its cousin bilberry, in Europe to help lower or regulate blood sugar in diabetics. Blueberry leaves have no known toxicity, and can be used for long periods of time on a regular basis.

Harvesting: Small leafy twigs can be gathered any time the plant holds healthy full-grown leaves—usually May through October. Pick the twiggy branches along the outside of the plant, and bundle in small batches to dry. Hang the bundles upside down in an airy place out of the sun. When leaves are dry and crumbly to the touch, strip them off the twigs, and store in an airtight container.

Dosages: Pour 1 cup of boiling water over 1–2 tablespoons of dried leaves, and let steep for 20 minutes or until cooled to body temperature. For urinary tract infections and gout, use 1 cup of strained tea three times daily. For elevated blood sugar associated with diabetes, 1 cup of tea before morning and evening meals can be taken on a regular basis.

FROM THE AUTHOR'S JOURNAL
JULY 15

Close by in the back field a deer is feeding. She has been there for as long as I've been up—10 minutes or so. She lowers her head to browse, tail wagging at the bugs, and makes few sounds. From 20 feet away I hear nothing except one soft huff of grass crushed for every step. She lowers her head to eat, then raises it, ears alert, eyes glittering. She freezes, then relaxes to browse again.

The doe moves a little, following the trail of whatever tender thing it is she eats, and slowly as the light increases in the sky, she moves in the direction of the woods without hurry. Her white tail flags behind her. As the sky turns pink and blue, the shadows lessen and she moves toward the apple trees, walking more than feeding now. It is close to 5 AM when her brown back is all I can follow through the fruit trees. Then she is out of sight.

Everything is damp as I follow her track to the pear tree. Along the way, chickweed is matted in the grass. I stop to pick some, looking around while I work for deer signs. I wonder if she ate some chickweed. It is tender, and I chew some as I gather it. Some of the tops are broken off, but the mower could have done that weeks ago. I finish in the field, lonely without the deer, and walk down the road that has puddles in it from last night's shower. At the roadside, raspberry leaves flutter. When I step into the brush to check the tansy for flowers, raspberries hang in the new sun, and I pick some and snack on them.

At Weeks's farm, the cattle are up and feeding in the field. One cow with a baby stops to stare at me while its calf butts against her udders, nursing. Down Big Sandy, the roadside is lush with blueberry bushes. Some of the berries are ripe, and I pick them to eat while I walk. There are branches where no berries grow, and I decide to start gathering my blueberry leaf supply for this season. I pick off leafy twigs 6 inches long or so and bundle them, eating while I work.

This feels so good to me, so simple and right—slow looking and slow picking, one easy branch after another. It makes such sense. Out in the field, the cows feed, too, and I wonder if they feel like I do, content and calmed. A little wind lifts the leafy branches, and lifts my hair. I walk home with the day's harvest, grateful for the land that takes care of me. I've had a free breakfast, visited with a neighborhood doe, and gathered the day's herb all in a little bit of stolen time before the day starts. What could be nicer?

Experiences with Blueberry

My favorite way to use blueberry leaves is as a tea to help control blood sugar in diabetics. Such a simple thing, a cup or two daily of blueberry leaf tea. But it works. Several years ago I met a woman on an herb walk whose mother had had diabetes for years. The daughter told her mother about blueberry leaves, and her mother spent the summer gathering the herb. In fall, after one month of using blueberry leaves, her blood sugar had fallen back to within normal limits, and remained there. Now she's a convert, and gathers blueberry leaves every year.

St. John's-wort
Hypericum perforatum

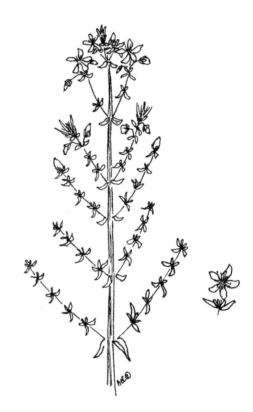

Reflections: I walk the development road today, not to pick anything, just to hike and look. The cleared areas are not clear anymore. A million now green things have gotten taller, and the bare soil is covered with a thick carpet, glittery with dew. New growth in some places is taller than I am. Underneath bright leaves, raspberries dangle, and I pick a few to eat. St. John's-wort pokes up in little clumps nearby, so I gather an armful of the flowery stems to take with me. On the way home, mist has settled over the wet land and I walk through clouds.

Description: St. John's-wort is a common wildflower of fields and roadsides. It may also be found in transitional zones between field and forest.

The leaves are bright green, up to 2 inches long, narrow and oblong. They occur frequently along stiff stems, growing in alternate directions. The leaves are distinctive, making it easy to recognize the plant even when not in flower. The smooth-margined leaves are marked with tiny translucent dots that show clearly when the leaf is held up to the sun or light. The stems are highly branched, and plant height is up to 2^1/$_2$ feet.

St. John's-wort flowers are bright yellow with many stamens. The blossoms have five petals, each having black dots along its ragged margin. Flowers occur in clusters atop the branched stems and are up to 1 inch wide. St. John's-wort flowers throughout the summer and into early fall.

The fruit is a small, dark, reddish brown capsule that may occur on a plant while it still bears blossoms.

Medicinal Uses: St. John's-wort is mildly sedative and antispasmodic. It can be used for anxiety, depression, general irritability, seasonal affective disorder (SAD), and insomnia. In depressions, it works best if the depressive symptoms are situational. St. John's-wort can be helpful when added to other herbs for menopausal changes, where it will help alleviate tension and mood swings.

St. John's-wort is also anti-inflammatory and astringent, and can be used externally for new bruises and sprains. An oil made of the fresh plant can be applied to the affected area as soon as possible after the initial injury. The oil can also be helpful in treating sunburn, wounds, or skin irritations, where it will help to relieve swelling and inflammation, tone affected tissues, and reduce the chances of scarring.

St. John's-wort is also mildly diuretic, and the plant can be used in minor bladder infections or irritations where there is difficulty with urination. It is also antiviral, and can be used in the first stages of a viral infection.

Harvesting: The aerial parts should be cut in summer and processed soon after gathering, since fresh-plant preparations are most effective. A fresh-plant tincture can be made, or an extracted oil can be prepared by covering the fresh, chopped whole plant with a vegetable oil. Add a little vitamin E oil or tincture of benzoin to keep the oil from getting rancid, and set the jar in the sun or in a warm place for 2 weeks. After this time, pour off the oil and store.

St. John's-wort contains an active principle, hypericin, which produces a deep red coloring, so both the oil and the tincture will be dark red. The blossoms can be used as a natural dye for wool or other fibers.

Dosages: The fresh-plant tincture can be taken three times daily in doses of 30 drops each. For a tea, use 1–2 tablespoons of fresh plant material per cup of boiling water, steep 20 minutes, and drink three times daily. The dried plant can also be used for tea or to make a tincture.

Externally, the oil is applied soon after injury and then frequently throughout the day. A poultice can also be made by moistening cotton or gauze with the oil, tincture, or tea and applied directly to the injured area. The poultice can be left on overnight.

CAUTION: St. John's-wort may cause photosensitivity in some light-skinned people. In this case, those likely to react should avoid long exposure to sunlight when taking the herb.

FROM THE AUTHOR'S JOURNAL
JULY 20

Early this morning I am up thinking of six thousand things I have to do in the next few days. To escape, I go out to feed the birds and then for a walk. The air is damp and coolish, and the grass is full of dew. As I walk, my mind begins to let go and my body relaxes.

Down at Weeks's farm, the cows lie close to the stone wall, sleeping. One cradles its huge head on another's solid back. Flies decorate her face, and her tail swings absently. I tiptoe by them. It is only 5 AM and the farmer won't be out to milk for another hour. They shift and glance at me, change positions, and settle again.

Down by the development road, I stand looking along the grassy banks to see what's come up, and I am amazed at how much new growth there is. Raspberry canes seem to cover everything. Underneath the canes, leaves of wild strawberry cluster along the ground. The white flower heads of bristly stemmed sarsaparilla poke up and I trace them to their main stem, remembering I want to gather some of the roots this fall.

I taste a few raspberries. They are sweet and ripe so I decide to look for more. On the older canes, leaves are dried and brown and shrunken, but the red stems hold lots of fruit. I make my way through the prickly new shoots to pick. I eat some berries and put more in my head net, using it like a bag. Farther down the road, the soil is damp, and I sink when I walk on it. Deer tracks are deep and clear. Cattail stands like tall green fans, spreading along the little streambank. I wish I could walk in farther, follow the waterway to the lake like the animals must. Instead, I stick to the road and find more berries, and my bag fills up fast.

In a nearby clearing, the yellow flowers of St. John's-wort catch my eye. I walk down to see them, into the green that gets lusher with each step. The flowers are full open and no seedpods have started to form. The leaves are so pretty and distinctive that I have learned to recognize this herb even when there are no flowers yet. I pluck one leaf now, hold it up to my eye, and look through tiny holes that dot the leaf. I see white clouds and the tops of trees clearly. Blue sky winks at me. I pack up my berries and walk home, watching the world through a St. John's-wort leaf.

Kitchen Notes

At home, I make a St. John's-wort oil to use for bruises and sprains. The herb, flowers and all, gets chopped up into a jar, with olive oil poured over it. Within a few days, the oil has turned a deep, bloodred—quite a surprising color from those green leaves and yellow blossoms! It makes me want to try using St. John's-wort as a dye for basket materials. Maybe it would produce the same, dark tint.

Experiences with St. John's-wort

Last fall when I tore a muscle in my leg, I used St. John's-wort oil externally. The effect was subtle, but I think it helped. I've used the tincture, too, mainly in formulas for nervousness and tension along with other herbs for the nervous system. The action was mild, but dependable, and now I make sure to gather St. John's-wort every year.

SELF-HEAL
Prunella vulgaris

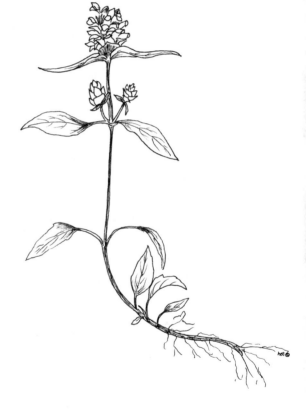

Reflections: I stand at the entrance to the woods and just sniff at the air and look around me, then close my eyes and take deep breaths. When I open them, there is self-heal at my feet—lots of it. It turns the grasses purple much as the violets did in early spring. I think how nice it is to see it so healthy and strong and how nice it will be to take home a part of this beautiful place.

Description: A common wild-flower of fields and roadsides, self-heal, also known as heal-all, is a Mint family member that tends to grow in clumps up to 1 foot in height. It often grows in lawns and will flower there even when cut at a height of 2–3 inches. It will grow in a variety of conditions and can be found in moist soil of woodland transitional zones or in dry fields.

Self-heal has opposing leaves that grow in pairs along a square stem. The leaves are lance or oval shaped, 1–3 inches long, and can have smooth or slightly toothed margins. The lower leaves may have longer stalks than the uppermost leaves.

The purple or violet blossoms are about $1/2$ inch long and occur on a head that is generally longer than it is wide. The upper lip of the flower is arched, and the lower lip is fringed and drooping. Dried brown flower heads are easy to spot after the flowers fade and often seem to be more elongated than the blossom itself.

Medicinal Uses: Self-heal is a gentle herb with mild action. It is astringent, which makes it useful for mild diarrhea in tea form. As a gargle or wash, self-heal can help reduce inflammation and soothe tissues of sore throats and gums. Added to other herbs in a tea taken during the first stages of a cold, it will help reduce mild fevers and the queasy feelings that accompany an illness. Externally, it can be crushed and used as a poultice for minor scratches, wounds, insect bites, or bruises.

Harvesting: Gather aerial parts just as the plant comes into flower. Be sure to gather only plants that are in true flower or are budding. Avoid those that have bloomed and bear dried brown flower heads. Bundle stems using rubber bands, and hang the plant upside down to dry. When fully dry, store in an airtight container for later use. Being a mildly active herb, self-heal will probably lose its usefulness after 6 months or so, so it is a good idea to check for scent and taste, and discard whatever seems lifeless after that time period.

Dosages: Use 1–2 tablespoons of dried plant to 1 cup of boiling water for a tea and steep 15–20 minutes. The tea can be drunk three or four times daily or used as a gargle or wash. The clean, fresh, crushed plant can be applied externally to minor skin irritations, held in place with gauze, and removed after 15 minutes or so. A new poultice can be reapplied if desired. The dried plant can also be used in a salve for the same skin irritations.

A light rain falls. Everything is green and wet outside. Water slides down leaves and drips onto the sodden earth. It runs in rivulets down the bigger hills I walk and stands in puddles all along the road. The rain is a persistent mist that has fallen through the night, and the morning is good, and close, and restful. The garden will be happy. And all the little streams should fill, making it easier for the animals in the forest who have needed water.

Jewelweed has sprouted in the ditches. Now that it is bigger, I recognize its leaves. There are no blossoms yet, so it's not really ready to pick. The stems are bluish and look juicy, and the leaves stand straight out to the sides of the plant. There are several roadkills, all frogs. Some are squished flat, and some are just limp, upside down. At the base of the big hill, I step into the woods. In early spring I would walk into a clearing farther back and just lie on the ground. There were lots of animal signs. A week or so ago, I saw a deer here, and nearby, a bear crossed the road and entered these woods. Lately the grass and brush are waist high, so I haven't been in.

As I look around, there is more self-heal here than I've seen anywhere. Its purple flowers sparkle in the morning's mist. I gather some to use for the beginnings of colds or coughs or sore throats and avoid a fat yellow slug trying to hide on one leaf. Some of the leaves show his shiny trail, and I avoid them, too.

I walk on home with the day's harvest in hand, and see the cows near the fence at Weeks's farm. One steer, one cows and a baby bull. I get closer and the steer sniffs at me. His square, even teeth show as his lip raises. His nose is covered with flies that move as he does. I offer him a sprig of self-heal, he sniffs at it but won't taste. He has a mouthful of grass already. I walk on, wishing them luck with the flies, promising to bring apples next time.

Kitchen Notes

At home, I put the self-heal down and three tiny insects race across the table. They are little see-through things, and scurry about wondering where they are. Across the folded newspaper, across the scuffed wood tabletop, across the bag they got here in. Poor things—I've changed their reality.

The same thought hit me as I stood harvesting self-heal in the bit of woods this morning. Self-heal is abundant here. Even in the close mown grass I can find it. And yet, when I pull up even one plant, I change things. I am amazed at my impact. I insert myself rudely into a natural world and alter everything. Next year self-heal may not grow where I have gathered it. The tiny bugs who race around on the table wondering where they are will not go home. Even if I place them back outside, they are uprooted and everything has changed for them. How dare I change the world? How dare I think that because I am big and mobile and they are small or rooted I can decide their fate? How dare I make things relative? There is no relative. Everything is a life, whole, belonging to itself. How dare I insert myself so aggressively into the lives of the field or woods and wield my will?

I dare because I do, I guess. I am just another species, making my way in the world, making one tiny ripple in the sea of my surroundings. I capture the little bugs on the newspaper and brush them onto the grass outside the door. I dry the self-heal that sometime this year will be used to help people who will then go about their lives, giving and changing and someday dying, to become dust again and fertilize some other woods or field or plot of ground. In the meantime, it's all life. It's what I choose, as carefully as I can, and it moves and changes and grows. I scoop up one more tiny bug to put outside, and get on with my chores.

LOBELIA
Lobelia inflata and species

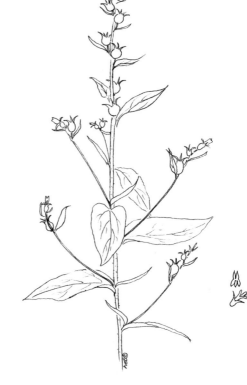

Reflections: Along the edges of the woods, lobelia looks terrific. Each branched stem is tipped with lavender blossoms and is full of puffy seedpods. Under the tallest plant, at the mouth of an overgrown field, a little garter snake coils protectively, watching me. He tastes the air and my scent, feints an attack, then settles down to wait. His whole, silky body expands and settles until, finally, he is only a dark spot on the gray and sandy road.

Description: *Lobelia* species are wildflowers common to roadsides, open woods, and fields, including lawns. While all species have medicinal value, *Lobelia inflata* is the most potent. It is also the one most commonly used in herbal tradition, and will therefore be described here.

The leaves of *Lobelia inflata,* commonly known as Indian tobacco, are alternate, oval shaped, and softly toothed. The leaves are up to 2 1/2 inches long, and are bright, light green in color. The central stem is often much branched in taller plants, with side branches sprouting from leaf axils. Plant height varies from 3 inches in lawns to up to 3 feet in undisturbed areas.

The flowers are tiny, about $1/4$ inch in length, and are pale lavender in color. The flower has two lips, the top one divided into two lobes and the bottom lip into three sharply pointed lobes typical of all *Lobelia* species. Flowers occur at the terminal ends of the stem and branches in summer through fall. The fruit is an inflated seed capsule formed from the blossom calyx, and after flowering the plant can be recognized by the many pale capsules along the stem and branches.

Medicinal Uses: Lobelia is antispasmodic and expectorant, and it is a respiratory stimulant in small doses (see Caution). Lobelia, used appropriately, can be helpful in asthma and bronchitis where it will stimulate expectoration and relax the respiratory tissues. It can also be used as an addition to other herbs in treating respiratory infections, where it will act to relieve a cough.

Harvesting: Gather aerial parts throughout the growing season as long as leaves are still healthy and green. Seeds are also medicinal, so if the plant has inflated seed capsules along the stem but few flowers, it can still be gathered and used. Bundle stems at the bottom, and hang to dry; or make a fresh-plant tincture. The dried plant tends to weaken quite a bit, and dosages become hard to predict, so tincturing the fresh plant is a good idea.

Dosages: Use 5–15 drops of the fresh-plant tincture three or four times daily. A tea of the dried plant can be made, using $1/2$ teaspoon of the plant to 1 cup of boiling water and steeping for 10 minutes. Chewing a small leaf of the fresh plant can sometimes bring relief in asthma.

CAUTION: Lobelia can be a toxic herb in doses other than those recommended. It is depressive to the central nervous system, and it is emetic, producing nausea and violent vomiting. An overdose can lead to convulsions and spinal cord depression. It should not be used without the supervision of a licensed practitioner.

I start out when there is no color in the sky yet. It's another damp morning, and my shoes are wet by the time I get to the road. The fields are full of mist, and full of the webs of tiny spiders called funnel weavers. The webs must be there all the time, but I only see them when it's early and damp, when dew turns them silvery gray.

I am out to gather lobelia. Two days ago I saw it for the first time this summer. Even though I've been looking for it, and think I know its leaves, it seems to be invisible to me until the tiny flowers appear. Yesterday, across from the lake where I gathered pipsissewa, lobelia grew all along the edges of the forest. It was tall, with lots of flowers, so it has been growing for some time. Seeing it there, I ran home to search the lawn. I've checked before and found nothing, but in the past week we've had lots of rain. And sure enough, one small plant stood neighbor to the sprouting Queen Anne's lace and new grass. I decided that lobelia must be in the woods, too, so today I'm out to look for it.

I take a new road that juts off down the hill. Along the roadside lobelia stands tall, even poking through the gravelly sand laid down for the road's foundation. For some reason, the plants that stand nearest the road are biggest. Maybe they get more sun. I pick the tallest plants and some shorter ones, pinching them off above a group of leaves, and leaving the roots intact. It can't be easy to grow in this sandy soil. If I leave some plants here there'll be more for next year.

The road dwindles into woods that are shadowy and wet. Bugs attack me and I pull up my hood and wear a head net for a while. In the middle of the path, more lobelia grows. It is shorter here, more shaded than its relatives outside that catch the sun all day long. Other things crowd along the little path, too—sorrel, self-heal, wild strawberry. In a clearing, the scent of raspberries makes me turn around to see them dangling from every thorny branch. I pick more lobelia as I walk, and finally, when the path juts off toward home, I've got a huge bouquet. The scalloped leaves with tiny lavender flowers and puffy seedpods are pretty enough for a table setting.

I put my finger to my mouth, and the familiar reaction begins—a tingling that's so intense it's almost uncomfortable. It stays in my throat for the 10 minutes it takes me to get home. Such a powerful effect from such a delicate-looking plant always amazes me.

Kitchen Notes

At home now, the beginnings of lobelia tincture set on the table, looking like an undersea jungle. In just the 5 minutes or so since I poured alcohol over it, the liquid is greenish and the lavender flowers are see-through. The color changes second by second. Seedpods float near the top like puffed up jellyfish. And now the tincture glows, translucent green. So much magic in one little jar is entrancing. I sit and watch for a while, and then I put the jar away.

Experiences with Lobelia

Last year I used lobelia a lot, in tiny doses. It went into the formula for my daughter's asthma. I used it, too, along with other herbs in formulas I made for seizure disorders. And I put it, in very small doses, in formulas for spasmodic coughs in winter. When I find it in the lawn these days, I let it stay, and circle it with the mower, wishing it luck. It's nice to have our very own supply so close at hand.

TANSY
Tanacetum vulgare

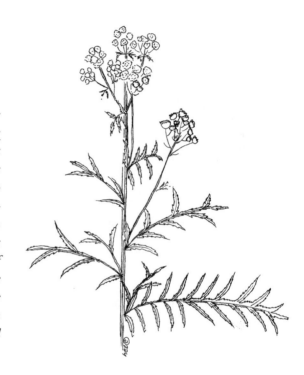

Reflections: At Big Sandy the blueberries are ripe and I pick some to eat. They are all wet with dew. While I work, birds settle in the branches next to me. Tansy that is full of yellow flowers threads through the blueberry bushes and leans toward the sun. I pick a few of the flowery stems to take home. Raindrops held on the leaves trickle down my arm and I shake the plants and bundle them.

Description: Tansy is a tall, yellow-flowered perennial of old gardens, now escaped and at home in sunny spots along roadsides and in fields. Tansy was often planted in dooryards and around the entrances to homes as it was thought to be helpful in preventing ants and other insects from entering the house.

The leaves are hightly divided, and leaflets are long and sharply toothed. Tansy leaves may grow up to 8 inches in length and occur along the stem alternately. When crushed, the leaves emit a strong scent. The plant may attain a height of 4 feet in favorable locations.

Tansy blossoms are simple heads of yellow disk flowers about $1/4$ to $1/2$ inch wide. The flower when mature looks like the head of a small daisy, minus the white ray petals. Blossoms appear on the plant mid-summer through fall.

Medicinal Uses: The leaves and blossoms of tansy have a limited use. Its primary current use is as a vermifuge and anthelmintic—that is, as an aid in killing and expelling intestinal parasites such as round-worms or tapeworms.

Tansy was at one time used as an emmenagogue to help regulate the female reproductive system and to stimulate the menstrual flow. However, it is believed to have been a cause of miscarriage in some cases and therefore should be avoided in pregnancy. Tansy also has some reputation as an herbal bitter and in the past was used to stimulate the digestive process and to ease colic and intestinal gas problems.

Harvesting: Gather the blossoms and leaves when the plant is in full bloom. Flowering stems may be cut about halfway down the plant, and the cut ends bundled and hung to dry. When moisture has evaporated, cut the plant into small pieces and store for later use.

Dosages: For intestinal parasites, make an infusion of tansy leaves and blossoms using 1 tablespoon of herb to 1 cup of boiling water. Steep for 10 minutes, and drink twice daily for 2 weeks. If any adverse symptoms occur, stop taking the tea.

CAUTION: Tansy contains oils that can be toxic in large doses, and it should never be taken for long periods of time or during pregnancy. Doses should be carefully regulated, and supervision by a licensed physician should be sought.

It's a wet, wet morning. We've had another rain and today the mist is so thick it feels like a cool steam bath. Last night the fields were misty, too, and as the sun went down, clouds were rose colored. The mist in the fields caught and held color until everything blushed pure magic. This early morning, moonlight streamed in my bedroom window and when I knelt to look out, the full moon gleamed through a halo of thick fog.

I am out with a bag to pick tansy. Leaving home, I take off my shoes. The grass is long and wet. Where I walk, wild chamomile is crushed and scents the air with pineappley fragrance. There are puddles on the road. Across from the house, robins stand on the fence and dive for worms the rain has flushed out of the soil.

Down the road at Weeks's field the cows are sleeping, mist settled on them like a blanket. Several lie together, heads cradled on each other. One rests his head on the wet grass and another is awake but drowsy. I try to move quietly past, but they sense me and shift, and move their heads to sniff at the air.

Near the stone wall I check on the tansy and find the first flower heads. These poor plants have to do all their growing in the shade of the maple trees. Today, tansy leans with the rain's weight. Its leaves are droopy, and four to five plants bear tiny, sunny blossoms just beginning to show color. A few days ago, down Porter Road, I passed a friend's house and saw tansy in lush, full growth. She has planted it near the dooryard steps to keep ants out of the house, but tansy can spread and take over, so I usually just gather it in the wild.

Today, these plants are ready to harvest. The pretty leaves are heavy with rainwater, and I blow crystal drops from the flowers. I pick a few of the stems and bundle them to take home for tea. Finally the sun comes up through the thick fog. Its edges are clear and its color mellow— much like the full moon this early morning. Tansy springs up now, its rain weight lessened by the coming sun. By the time I leave for home, it stretches full tilt out of the shadows, reaching for the light.

Kitchen Notes

I bundle the tansy to hang. The stems are slightly ridged and smell sweet and clean, a little like soap. When I crush a ruffly leaf, the odor is intensely aromatic. Maybe it's the odor the ants don't like. I taste a bit of leaf but then spit it out. The bitterness lingers on my tongue for a while, a not-very-nice sort of taste. Soon, the room has filled with the intense scent and I decide I like the fragrance better than the taste.

BLUE COHOSH
Caulophyllum thalictroides

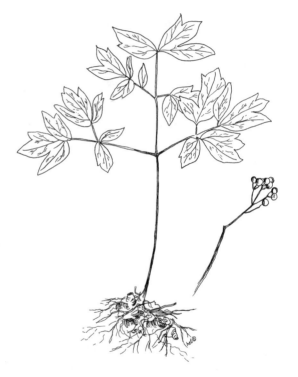

Reflections: Near the place where I rest, a little stream moves without a ripple, slowly, as if it's tired. Purple pickerel weed and white and yellow pond lilies stand in bloom. The shallow water is lush with red and green algae. I shift the blue cohosh to a bag and several mallards take flight, startled. Sun beats down on the water, but the shadows of the woods keep me cool.

Description: Blue cohosh is a woody plant found in rich moist woods. Although it is not abundant, it often grows in large populations.

The leaves are deeply and irregularly lobed. They are compound, divided into numerous leaflets, with each leaflet up to 3 inches in length. Leaves occur alternately along the stem. The foliage is decorative, with each leaflet having two to five deep, irregular, pointed lobes. The leaflets are stalkless. Plant height is up to 3 feet.

Blue cohosh flowers are $^1/_2$ inch wide and have six small petals inside six larger sepals. They range in color from yellowish green to purplish brown and occur spring to early summer. The blossoms grow in loose clusters at the ends of branches. Stems and branches are somewhat woody.

The fruit is a dark, dusky blue seed that resembles a blueberry. The berries occur atop small inflated stalks appearing green in late summer and then deepening in color as the weather cools. Berrylike seeds remain on the plant through early winter and maintain their deep blue color.

Medicinal Uses: Blue cohosh is known as an emmenagogue, a uterine tonic, and an antispasmodic. It was used by the Native American women during the last stages of pregnancy as a preparation for labor and delivery. It was especially favored if labor was long and the mother became exhausted. Although described by some herbalists as a preventive for miscarriage, it should probably not be taken until the last month of pregnancy.

As an emmenagogue, blue cohosh can stimulate the menstrual flow and can be used in menstrual irregularity where it can help regulate the flow. In the case of late menstrual periods, blue cohosh can aid in promoting menses. It is helpful in painful periods where its antispasmodic action helps to relieve cramps. It can also be used in endometritis. In menopause, it is helpful when there is pain with menstruation.

Harvesting: The root and rhizome are the parts used. These can be dug up in the fall after foliage has begun to die back. The cleaned roots can be tinctured right away, or they can be sliced and spread out to dry. The dried roots can be tinctured later or used as tea. Blue cohosh contains compounds that are not particularly soluble in water, so the tincture form is best.

HARVESTING CAUTION: Blue cohosh is a rare or at-risk plant in many of the areas to which it is native. Contact your state environmental agency or local herb guild to determine its status.

Dosages: Take 5–15 drops of tincture three times daily. If using the tea, place 1 teaspoon of dried root in water, simmer 10–15 minutes, and drink three times daily.

CAUTION: Blue cohosh should be avoided during the first two trimesters of pregnancy.

FROM THE AUTHOR'S JOURNAL
JULY 29

On the way home from camping in the mountains, I stop at an old farmhouse that offers perennial plants for sale. I'm looking for elecampane to put in my garden at home, and haven't seen it yet. This place doesn't have it either, but I walk through the gardens and see blue cohosh, another herb I've been wanting to find. The owner doesn't have enough to sell, but a neighbor offers me some of hers, so we trek out to her back woods to dig some up.

We walk back along a path and cross a wide clearing. In the middle of the field, sedges grow where water collects when the neighboring stream backs up. We see red clover having its second growth spurt, and little lavender lobelias, and some St. John's-wort and yarrow. All of this field was cut recently, but has grown up again to knee-high in some spots. Near the woods, there are trails made by deer and bear. The bear has two cubs this year, and is hard-pressed to keep them fed.

As we enter the woods, a wide path has been trampled. Uprooted shrubs and overturned rocks show where the bear hunted for grubs with her babies. Just beyond the bear litter, blue cohosh stands, about knee-high. It is full of pretty leaves, and bears round greenish berries starting to turn blue. They color the place up, as dusky as ripe blueberries, but larger.

I pick a likely plant and start to dig with a trowel, but the roots are firmly planted and the trowel handle snaps, so I finish the job with my hands. The root has lots of snaky rootlets that spread out in all directions. One plant that looks tiny has a large root that leads to fatter roots all knotted together. The root lengths are smooth and have just-visible ridges along them, and in some places roundish nubs where perhaps some other sprout will start soon.

I dig up a few more plants to take home, then walk back through the woods. At a swampy spot near the forest edge, the soil is black and sticky where water from a nearby stream turns it to clay. The soil is printed with deer tracks that cover each other in layers, a sure sign of a deer wallow. Animals must come to coat themselves with mud to keep the bugs away. There is a sweet and musky scent in the air, not the fetid smell I sometimes notice when animals are frightened. They must feel protected here. I back out quickly, hoping my human scent won't startle them, and take my bag of roots home.

Kitchen Notes

When I pull the blue cohosh from the bag, very round berries fall from some stems and roll around on the tabletop. Soil gets cleaned from larger roots under running water. The thinnest rootlets curl about each other and around my fingers as I work. The cleanest roots get chopped into a jar with alcohol poured over them. The little jar will set in the herb cabinet for a few weeks to make a tincture. The plants that are left over I'll put back in the woods where they can establish a new home. Then I'll have my own supply close by, and a new and beautiful inhabitant for the local woods.

Experiences with Blue Cohosh

Last year I offered blue cohosh to a friend who was in the final month of pregnancy. She had gone through two very long labors with previous children, and she and her midwife wanted to try blue cohosh to make her work easier. She started taking the herb a week or so before her due date, and managed to deliver on time. The labor was still long, but easier and quicker than before, and she felt that the blue cohosh had something to do with that.

VALERIAN
Valeriana officinalis

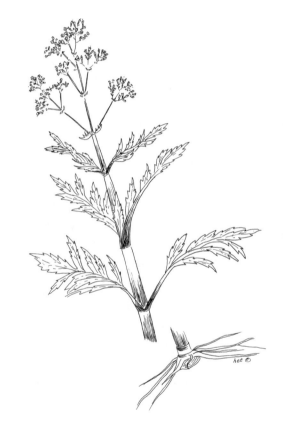

Reflections: In the 100 degree heat, I kneel in the brush and dig hands deep into hard soil, following rootlets to a main stem. I have tumbled into the ditch twice already. My arms are sticky and itching, and there is soil caked in all the creasy places of my skin. Suddenly the soil breaks loose. The deep, earthy, unforgettable scent of valerian drifts up, and I know all the hard work was worthwhile.

Description: Valerian is a tall, pretty plant often used in wild-flower gardens. It was planted in early gardens, and now is naturalized in many areas, being found along damp roadsides and in fields or meadows.

The leaves are deeply divided into numerous leaflets. The leaflets have smooth margins or may be slightly toothed or ragged looking at the tips. The deep divisions give the leaves a fernlike appearance. Leaf length is up to 10 inches. Leaves occur in opposing pairs out of a stiff, highly grooved, hollow stem. Plant height is up to 5 feet. The root is surprisingly small considering the plant's height, and the root has a deep woodsy-spicy scent that is evident when it is dug, persisting even in the fresh-root preparations. Dried roots tend to smell rank and musty.

Valerian's flowers are small, up to $1/4$ inch long, and occur in flattened, branched clusters at the top of the plant. Blossoms are fragrant and have five regular petals. They range in color from white to pinkish lavender. Valerian blooms in summer, although some blossoms may be found into the fall.

Medicinal Uses: Valerian is known chiefly for its sedative properties. It is also antispasmodic, hypnotic, and hypotensive. All these properties make valerian useful for anxiety and tension, where it will help to produce a relaxed state.

It can be helpful in a formula with other herbs for some seizure disorders, where it acts as an antispasmodic and helps calm the nervous system. Valerian helps to relax both skeletal and organ muscles, and it is useful in relieving many kinds of pain, from menstrual cramps to migraine headache. A preparation of valerian root is effective without producing druglike aftereffects.

As a muscle relaxant and hypnotic, valerian can also be used in insomnia, where, again, it does not leave a druglike dopiness as tranquilizers might. It is best taken shortly before bedtime and can be repeated as necessary. It does not have any reported toxicity.

Harvesting: Identify valerian carefully before digging. Another plant likely to be found in the same kind of habitat, with similar flowers and height, is water hemlock, which is highly toxic. Water hemlock has leaves divided into shorter, wider leaflets that are roughly and consistently toothed. The stems are often purple, especially near the base, and the root is not odorous, as is valerian root. It is a good idea to find valerian in summer when it is in full bloom and leaf material is available for identification, and mark each plant stem with bright twine. In the fall, return to these plants and gather only the ones that are marked.

When ready to harvest valerian, dig the root, and clean it thoroughly. Valerian should be prepared as a fresh-plant tincture because drying allows the formation of a compound that can cause depression if taken over a period of time. Slice the fresh, cleaned root into a jar, cover with alcohol, and set aside for two weeks. Then scoop out spent plant, strain tincture, and bottle to store. Valerian can also be dried to use as an occasional tea by slicing the root thinly and spreading out to dry on screens, baskets, or paper. Store when a piece snaps easily between your fingers.

Dosages: A tincture of valerian can be taken three times a day in doses ranging from $1/2$–2 teaspoons. If using valerian for pain, the dose can be repeated within half an hour if the first dose is not effective. When taking valerian for insomnia, take it about 20 minutes before bedtime. Again, the dose can be repeated if it does not seem effective within a half hour.

CAUTION: The dried-root preparation should not be taken on a regular basis as it can cause depression. This effect is not found in the fresh-root preparation.

FROM THE AUTHOR'S JOURNAL
AUGUST 5

It's too hot again. I can't stand to be still. I haven't unpacked the car from camping, but it's too hot to think about doing anything indoors. I wander around the house unable to settle, and decide to go get blueberries. Every year I buy some to add to the ones I pick for the freezer so we can have them year-round. At least driving will get me out of the house.

The trip to South Paris where the blueberries are sold is an hour's drive away, but at least the car is moving and makes a tolerable breeze. Still, I say a hundred times, "God, it's hot!"—with only myself to hear.

The dirt road I finally take climbs high along a mountain ridge. From here, every corner and curve of the valley below is visible. The next mountain cuts gently into this one, and the few houses on it are tiny specks. Today a haze hangs around the ridges.

Along roadsides I keep an eye out for whatever grows here. Some of the usual plants—evening primrose, and raspberry, and tangly blackberries—are visible. Something tall with an umbel-type flower is going to seed, and I drive slower, trying hard to see it. I think its leaves look familiar, and hope that it's the valerian I've been wanting to find. I decide to stop on my way back down the hill.

At the blueberry place, the farmer sits under a tree. Dusky, plump blueberries lie in shallow wooden trays stacked at angles on top of each other, in the shade, too. The farmer weighs out 40 pounds for me, and says to get them home and refrigerated right away. "One hundred degree is hard on the fruit," he says. Hard on us, too. Hard on everything.

Driving back down the steep hill, blueberry boxes are propped into the seat so they don't slide forward with the hill's slope. I drive slowly and seek out the scraggly heads of the plant I saw before. When I spot a few, I park on the roadside, and race over to see what they are. And sure enough, it looks like the valerian I've gathered in other states. I've never seen it in bloom, and these blossoms are half-gone, tiny, wind-blown flowers in a cluster. The leaves look familiar—deeply divided, with the tips of each leaf raggedly angled and blunt. Back at the car, I grab a shovel and then jump onto the hilly slope where the plant grows. I tap around to get a feel for where the roots would be, brush away grass and nearby plants with my hands. The plant's stem is slightly reddish near the base. I place the shovel and step on it, jump down hard when resistance is offered—and tumble into the ditch. Another try and the shovel sinks, and the answer wafts up to me in the air—the deep and heady scent of valerian root.

I tear up a small patch of earth and root, hold the root up to my nose, and sniff deeply. What a wonderful smell! This is the wrong time to gather valerian, though, so I gather just two plants—one to dry and one to put in the garden. In the next few days I'll come back to tie little bits of red yarn around the stems that stand here. Then, in the fall, I'll recognize it easily. For now, I'm just glad to have found it.

I put the tall plants in the back of the car, and put my shovel up. A few flower heads of valerian go on top of the blueberries. I catch sight of myself in the car window, and realize how grubby I am. Sweat and soil cake along my skin and bits of twiggy stuff are tangled in my hair. But I don't mind. I'm so glad to have found valerian, I don't mind at all. I ride now, eating hot blueberries with gritty hands, and sing to myself all the way home.

Experiences with Valerian

I first used valerian for occasional insomnia. Mostly I sleep just fine, but a few years ago, when I was working and going to school, stress had me waking in the middle of the night, unable to return to sleep. Then, I reached for valerian. I took it the first time, hopped back into bed with a magazine, read for a few minutes, and could actually feel my muscles starting to relax. By the time I turned out the light, my eyelids were heavy and I was half-dreaming already.

Last year when I tore a muscle in my leg, valerian was the first thing I took for pain. My daughter has used it, too, for a different problem. She developed a seizure disorder following a head injury, and decided to take valerian whenever she had a seizure aura. She hasn't had seizures for almost 10 years now, and only occasionally does she feel the need to take valerian anymore. Obviously, a physician must be consulted in such situations, but we really believe that the valerian was a useful part of the treatment.

MINT
Mentha species

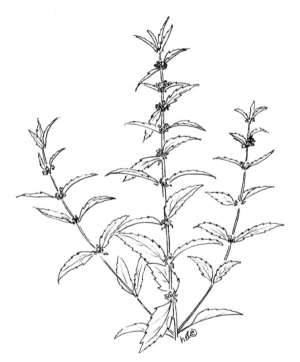

Reflections: New green growth has leapt up since the last time I was down this hill. As usual, the farther I walk, the quieter I feel. Near the bottom of the hill I stand still. Everything feels different—more peaceful. A breeze moves the leaves, and in trees nearby, birds play in and out of branches. The flash of a goldfinch moves in the shadows and I keep track of him with my eyes for a while. At the roadside, mint crowds, full of lavender flowers. I pick a few of the leafy stems and the intense scent drifts in the breeze.

Description: The mints are aromatic plants commonly identified by their square stems and opposing leaves. Numerous varieties of mint can be found in the wild, and often species will intermingle, making true identification difficult.

Wild mint, *Mentha arvensis,* the only native mint in the Northeast, can be found throughout the region. Leaves are up to 3 inches long and are very aromatic. The leaves taper at both ends and occur in opposing pairs along the square stem. Blossoms are tiny, up to $1/4$ inch long and $1/8$ inch wide, with four petals. The flowers grow only in the leaf axils, and occur on plants summer through fall. Wild mint frequents damp meadows and clearings where it can grow up to 2 feet in height.

Peppermint, *Mentha piperita,* has escaped from cultivated gardens and may be used medicinally. Leaves are generally between 1 and $2^1/2$ inches long and are oblong or lance shaped. They are sharply toothed and occur in opposing pairs along the square stem. Flowers are pink to lavender, about $1/5$ inch long, with four lobes. They grow in thick whorled terminal clusters. Peppermint blooms early summer through late fall. The plant will grow up to 3 feet in height and is commonly found in a number of habitats, such as ditches, around homes, and in wet fields. It generally prefers damp soil.

Spearmint, *Mentha spicata,* is another migrant from cultivation. It has the same pinkish lavender, four-lobed flower, but these grow on a terminal cluster that is long and tapered. The blossoms occur in midsummer. Spearmint is generally unbranched. Leaves are sessile, or stalkless. Like peppermint, spearmint grows in damp places.

Medicinal Uses: The mints are aromatic, antispasmodic, carminative, stomachic, and analgesic. These properties make it useful in treating stomach upsets and indigestion, and mint tea can be used after heavy or disagreeable meals to lessen nausea and cramping or bloating. Oil of peppermint has been used in the treatment of ulcerative colitis to aid in reducing spasms and pain. As an antispasmodic, the herb can also be useful in tension and anxiety, where it produces a relaxing effect and its aromatic scent is soothing. In addition, it can be used to relieve menstrual cramps, where it will help stimulate delayed menses, and ease cramps.

The mints are also diaphoretic, producing a mild sweat and therefore helping the body to reduce fever in a natural way. Mint is a good adjunct to any therapy for colds and flu for this reason.

Harvesting: Gather the aerial parts of the herb just as it starts to flower. Bundle into small batches by wrapping the stems with a rubber band. Hang upside down to dry in a shaded, aerated place. Check in a week or so, and when the plant is crisply dried, store in an airtight container out of the sun. Being high in volatile oils, mint is susceptible to loss of potency if stored improperly, so be sure to keep the jar well closed and away from heat or light.

Dosages: Use 1–2 tablespoons of the dried herb, and make an infusion by pouring 1 cup of boiling water over it, letting it steep for 15–20 minutes. Drink several times daily.

FROM THE AUTHOR'S JOURNAL
AUGUST 7

This morning I take my first walk here in a week, hunting for blackberries. In the mountains where I camped, they were ripe and sweet, and I am eager to have more. I carry a bag for berries, and bring a head net in case the deerflies are still bad. Last time I was down the development road, the low prickly vines of blackberries had green fruit on them, so today I'll check them out.

Down the unused path, the hill slopes steeply. At its base, the earth is swampy—black and wet—and a trickle of water moves through. Cattails are tall and topped with brown spikes. I squeeze one with my fingers, and it feels solid and slightly furry. Near a widening of the tiny stream, boneset grows. The stand of plants I saw last week is still blossoming.

These swampy places are so lush with growth, so full of variety. My eyes are pulled from one green thing to another. There is so much to see! I glimpse at something down low that I haven't noticed before; I can't decide what it is from here. It stands at the edge of the wettest place, and I decide to try to reach it.

Up over the hilly part is easy. Then the trees give way to swamp, to fallen logs that lie in the shallow and dark water. I squat low to hold onto branches or cattail leaves for balance. Low like this, I recognize plants I hadn't seen from the path. The green stuff that crowds around the rotten log beneath me is bugleweed, full of tiny white flowers. Lobelia stands tall here, in full and vigorous bloom.

I squish along farther, and reach the end of the log. Brown water surrounds me, and the water is covered with a low, aquatic growth that forms a green lace network. Up on the opposite bank that edges the water, the plant I noticed before grows in clumps. It is one step too far away, but I want to see it close up. I take a chance, step into the squish, and stretch one foot over to a small rock projecting out of the water. Now the plant is just barely within reach. A pinched leaf releases a strong, minty scent. I pop a leaf in my mouth, and fall backward, landing on the log. I decide to sit for a while, chewing on the mint leaf, and try to decide what species of mint this is. It tastes very strong, full of flavor. Little lavender flowers grow in the leaf axils, clustering around the stem in a circle. Maybe this is the *Mentha arvensis,* known in this area as water mint. Or maybe it's a mix of several species. In any case, I can gather some to use for tea.

I get up to try again, and balance on the little rock that pokes out of the water. One good leap takes me to the far bank, and there is more of the mint growing in small, low clumps alongside the stream. I gather several bunches and tuck them into my pack along with the grass samples and berries. Finally, I squish across logs again to dryer ground, and then to the road and home.

Experiences with Mint

Last year we used mint for all kinds of problems, and just for its good taste, too. Mint went into tea mixes when we had colds or flu. It helped to reduce fevers, and was soothing at the same time. It also helped when stomachs were upset after huge holiday meals. Hot mint tea was one of our favorite drinks on blustery winter days. And friends liked it so much we gave it, in pretty jars, as Christmas gifts—a little reminder of the earth's blessings.

BONESET
Eupatorium perfoliatum

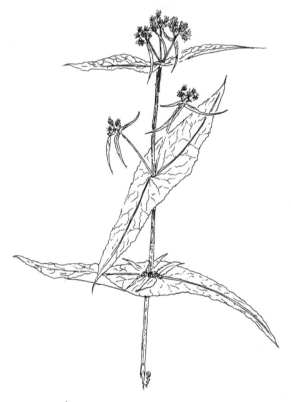

Reflections: Woods sounds lift around me. Coyotes sing in a distance, and I keep my eye out for bear. When I am in here, working quietly, I could be just another animal. I could stay and eat berries and chew the bitter boneset and drink from the stream. I could feed and work alongside the deer in the field and move quietly back into the woods before light comes.

Description: Boneset is a tall, coarse-leaved wildflower that appears summer through fall. The plant is found along damp roadsides, in ditches, and in moist meadows or waste places.

The leaves are lance shaped, with pointed tips. They are dark, glossy green on the surface, and slightly hairy underneath. The leaves occur in opposing pairs along the stiff stem. They are coarse in texture and appear wrinkly. Their most distinctive feature is the leaf bases, which completely surround the stem so that the stem appears to perforate the leaves (hence the Latin species name, *perfoliatum*). The leaf margins are roughly toothed and leaves are up to 8 inches long. The plant may attain a height of 4 feet.

Boneset flowers are tiny, up to $1/4$ inch long, and occur in flat-topped clusters at the top of the plant and side stems. Blossoms are white, grayish looking when opened, and are numerous. Boneset flowers midsummer through fall.

Medicinal Uses: Boneset is diaphoretic, diuretic, tonic, and antispasmotic. It will produce a sweat if drunk as a hot tea, thereby helping to relieve the fevers of colds and flu. Boneset is also helpful for relieving respiratory symptoms associated with a cold or influenza, where it acts as an antispasmodic, helping to relax membranes. In addition, boneset helps to relieve the deep bone or muscle aches that can accompany influenza. It is thought that boneset has some anti-inflammatory actions, and it is used for rheumatic and arthritic pain with some success. Taken as a cold infusion, boneset acts as a bitter tonic, stimulating digestive processes by its bitter taste.

Harvesting: Cut the plant just above ground level as it is beginning to form flower buds. Bundle at the stem bases, and hang to dry upside down for 1 to 2 weeks. When the leaves are crumbly, cut into $1/2$-inch pieces, and store in an airtight container. A fresh-plant tincture can be made of the plant soon after it is gathered and can be used in place of the infusion.

Dosages: Use 1 tablespoon of dried herb to 1 cup of boiling water for a hot infusion and steep 20 minutes. Drink $1/2$ cup of the tea every $1/2$–1 hour at the beginning of symptoms and then four times daily. For a cold infusion, soak the dried plant in water for 4–6 hours, using 1 tablespoon of dried herb to 1 cup of water, then strain, and drink in $1/2$ cup doses before meals. If using the tincture, take 30–40 drops every 4 hours. If taking the tincture as a bitter, mix in a little bit of water, and take 15–20 minutes before meals.

It's a funny kind of morning. Walking down the road as light steals into the sky, everything is rosy. Sun squints through a layer of cloud and turns the sky pink, and all the earth things, too, as I walk down the development road to get boneset. A large stand of it grows back in the wettish low ground where woods used to be.

Along the roadside there is scat from some small animal, full of blackberry seeds, and I wonder what animal passed here. Just at the bend in the road, boneset stands far back. There is no path leading to it, and the way in is barricaded by blackberry bushes and fallen logs and tree limbs, scattered when the area was cleared. The blackberry branches are full of fruit, the sweetest I've tasted this year, and the farther I go the better they get. My shirt gets snagged on brambles, and I wonder what animal can get to these innermost berries. Maybe birds.

Holding onto tiny trees for balance, I climb over logs and twigs and through prickly bushes until the brush gets lower and the ground wetter, over sandy soil that is covered with wetland grasses, and finally to the boneset. Most of it is in full flower. Its leaves are coarse and glossy on the top and true green. The flower buds are tiny, creamy white, and grow in flat-topped clusters. The blossoms that are fully open are dirty looking, like little bits of scraggly fluff. I pick a handful of the flowering stems. The plants that stand alone, I leave to grow bigger and seed.

Rains start, a funny rain. The mountain stands dark behind me, rising out of a grayish mist; up above, black and blue clouds cluster. Around their edges, blue sky shows, and in the east, the sun comes up clear and bright. I follow deer tracks along an easier path through the blackberry bushes, and get sprinkled all the way home by the teasing rain.

Kitchen Notes

In the kitchen, I chop up some of the plant to make a tincture. A few green mites and tiny white crab spiders scatter along the table, and I scoop them up and brush them out the back door to find new homes.

When I bring my fingers to my lips, they are bitter, like the boneset. Sometime soon, I'll gather more to dry for tea.

Later, sitting outside on the dooryard steps, I tie up the rest of the boneset bundles for drying. While I work, the feisty little dog who lives down the hill snuffs at the ground near the mailbox, eyeing me. Always, he dives and barks if I pass his house. The last time I was by, he followed me, barking and leaping and snarling, tiny thing that he is. I yelled and cursed and threatened and fended him off with a stick, and then finally laughed because the two of us were so funny. I think how good it would be if all my troubles were barking dogs, seeming fierce and determined, niggling at me, but really nothing more than a little game we play.

I pick up my bundles of boneset and go back inside, leaving the yard to the dog.

Experiences with Boneset

Several years ago I came down with an awful flu. I was so tired I could barely lift my eyelids. Every muscle and joint ached. A fever kept rising higher and other nasty cold symptoms were setting in. I had boneset on hand, a batch I had dried the previous summer, and had decided to try it as a tea. I made a strong infusion, settled back on the couch to take a huge swallow—and promptly spat it out! I thought I had poisoned myself. Surely, nothing good for me could taste so terrible! It took me half an hour to get through one cup of tea, but it worked. Within 2 hours the achiness was better, the cold symptoms were abating, and I felt human again. Maybe I got better because I was afraid of having to take more boneset. But I guess it doesn't matter—it worked!

MOTHERWORT
Leonurus cardiaca

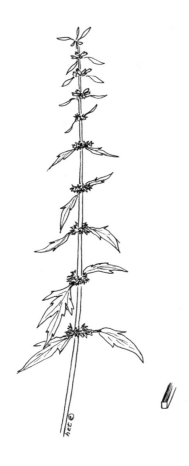

Reflections: I sit outside bundling motherwort, and glance up to see a red fox loping across the yard. She is small and thin, runs easily and in no particular hurry. She steps through the garden, sniffing at everything, and then into the back field where she races back and forth, chasing birds. She plays, leaping into the air, prancing one way or another, looking much like a cat. When she is tired of the field, she slips through the neighbor's fence and disappears, and I go back to the motherwort.

Description: Motherwort is a wildflower member of the Mint family. It thrives with moisture, but can do quite well in dryer areas, and it can be found in old fields, disturbed soil, and along roadsides. It produces seeds abundantly and often takes over an area where it grows.

Motherwort has a sharply squared stem and distinctly pointed, three-lobed leaves that occur in opposing pairs along the stiff, square stem. The leaves have deep lobes, usually three, that are sharply pointed. The lowest leaves may have five lobes. Leaf length may be up to 3 inches with the uppermost leaves getting gradually smaller. The plant can grow up to 5 feet in favorable locations.

The flowers are irregularly shaped and are up to only $1/2$ inch long and $1/3$ inch wide. The blossoms grow in a circle around the stem at the leaf axils and have five sepals with sharply pointed spines at their tips. The flower is two lipped, with the upper lip having two distinct lobes and the lower lip having three. The upper lip flares out over the lower and is slightly hairy. Blossoms appear summer through fall.

Medicinal Uses: Motherwort has two primary traditional uses. The first is indicated by its common name, "motherwort," referring to its use by women. The plant contains compounds that make it antispasmodic, emmenagogue, and sedative. These properties aid in relaxing smooth muscles and in regulating menstrual flow. The tea or tincture can be used in delayed menstruation and in PMS associated with anxiety, tension, and irregularity of flow. Motherwort can also be helpful as a tonic in menopause where cycles are becoming irregular and anxiety and irritability are factors. Motherwort can be especially helpful when menstrual irregularity is accompanied by heart palpitations or flutters of nervous origin.

Motherwort's Latin name, *Leonurus cardiaca,* indicates its other primary use. *Cardiaca* refers to the heart, and motherwort has been used traditionally as a heart tonic, where it works to strengthen and normalize heart action. It is mild and nontoxic. It is also helpful in palpitations that stem from nervousness and anxiety. Motherwort is weak in action and is a good adjunct to other, stronger herbs for heart problems or irregularity.

Harvesting: The aerial parts, including leaves, stems, and blossoms, is gathered as it is coming into bloom. Bundle the strong stems together at the cut bases, and hang the plant to dry in small batches in a well-ventilated place out of the sun. In one to two weeks, motherwort should be dry enough to store. A fresh-plant tincture can be made of the plant soon after gathering.

Dosages: A strong infusion can be made of motherwort, using 1–2 tablespoons of the dried herb to 1 cup of boiling water. Steep for 20 minutes, and drink three times daily. A tincture, made from either fresh or dried plant material, can be taken in doses ranging from ¹/₂ to 1 teaspoon three times daily. Start with a small dose, and increase if smaller doses do not seem effective.

FROM THE AUTHOR'S JOURNAL
AUGUST 16

Today, I'm harvesting motherwort. I walk over to a friend's house to gather herbs from her huge perennial garden. Lots of the things that grow here are medicinal. All the plants now are lush and strong, and I will gather whatever is ready. Catnip and comfrey get harvested. Valerian root can wait. Lobelia gets pulled up to dry, and in the greenhouse, passionflower is taking over a whole corner from top to bottom and gets cut back for a tincture.

Beside the cultivated plants, there are wild herbs that stand as weeds in the formal gardens. A fat-leaved chickweed sprouts around the compost, and I gather that. Evening primrose hasn't seeded yet, so it can wait. Back in the swampy woods near the stream that supplies water for the plants, bugleweed stands, but I let it stay, for I've already gotten some in the wild.

I check out the motherwort. I have gathered it before in fields, but this year I didn't find any. In the shaded garden, between other cultivated plants, motherwort is as tall as I am. It is just entering its flowering season. Some of the plants bear tiny purplish flowers that remind me of catnip blossoms. They grow in whorls at the leaf axils. Some of the flowers have begun to seed, too, and the seed is held in brownish sepals that are thorny and painful to touch. The leaves are what I remember best about motherwort—definite three-pointed lobes that grow on a tall, square stem.

There is lots of motherwort, here, and I bundle the plants to take home. The process is painful. The sharp sepals keep surprising me. Fifty or a hundred times I grab the plant the wrong way and get wounded. I have to remind myself of how useful motherwort is, and how much I'll like having it to use as a tonic.

By the time I get home, the bundles have attached themselves to each other, and when I pull them apart, some of the prickly seedpods fall everywhere and I step on them barefoot or sit on those that are stuck to my clothes. I have more bad things to say about motherwort, and I have to remind myself of how much I'll like it later.

Experiences with Motherwort

I've used motherwort a lot, for a range of different problems. It has gone into formulas for irregular periods, and for irritability with PMS. I've used it as an aid in menopause, and it seems to help calm frazzled nerves then. I've also used motherwort along with other herbs as a heart tonic, especially for people who experience palpitations with anxiety. Most of the time, I put motherwort in formulas along with other herbs, and find it gentle, mild, and reliable.

BLUE VERVAIN
Verbena hastata

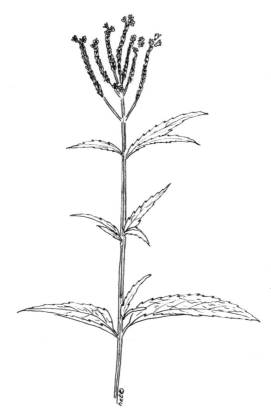

Reflections: The little stream is shallow now, water so low that the mossy tops of rock glisten in the sun. A breeze moves the leaves of the shading trees—maples, turning red already, and a few shrubby willows. Blue vervain shifts in the new wind, bright purple blossoms vibrant against the backdrop of sandy soil. I sit for a while and watch before I move on to harvest.

Description: A number of vervains can be used medicinally. The vervain of herbal tradition is *Verbena hastata,* commonly known as blue vervain. Blue vervain prefers moist soils of thickets, streambeds, roadsides, and meadows, and can be found along the seashore. The species is often planted as an ornamental in perennial gardens.

The leaves are lance shaped and grow 4 to 6 inches long. The margins are sharply toothed and the leaves are stiff, with a coarse texture. They occur in opposing pairs along the stiff, squared stem, and have short stalks. Plant height is up to 6 feet tall in optimal conditions, although is often seen about knee-high.

The blossoms of blue vervain are deep bluish lavender in color and occur in numerous terminal spikes atop a single stem. The flowers often appear sparse, since only a few open at a time, and seeds and buds may appear on the same flower spike. Flowers have five petals and are up to $^1/8$ inch wide. Blue vervain blooms in summer through fall.

Medicinal Uses: *Verbana hastata* and all its relatives have a range of medicinal properties that make them useful for a variety of complaints. The herb is known as a nervine, or nerve tonic, and it is sedative and antispasmodic. These attributes make it useful in anxiety and nervousness, where it acts to soothe and relax the nervous system. It is also helpful in insomnia and in the upset stomach that accompanies anxiety in some people. Blue vervain is especially useful for children who are restless when ill, but have a hard time settling down to recuperate.

Blue vervain is also diaphoretic and will help reduce a fever by producing a sweat. Combined with its other properties, the diaphoretic action makes vervain a helpful adjunct to therapies for children (or adults) who are coming down with a cold or flu. It can help reduce fever and at the same time work to relax and soothe nerves, thereby promoting the rest needed for the recovery process.

Harvesting: Cut aboveground stems when the plant is just starting to flower. Bundle in small batches at the bases, and hang upside down to dry. When leaves are brittle, remove flower spikes and leaves, and cut thinner top stems into small pieces. Discard any stem parts that seem woody. Store plant parts until ready to use. A fresh-plant tincture can also be made soon after gathering the herb, or a dried-plant tincture can be prepared later.

Dosages: When taking verbena as a tea, make an infusion using 1 tablespoon of dried herb to 1 cup of boiling water. Steep for 20 minutes, and drink three times a day. For children, use $^1/2$ teaspoon of herb to 1 cup of water, and give $^1/2$ cup of the tea three times daily. If taking the tincture, 30 drops, or $^1/4$ teaspoon, may be taken three times daily.

If using for children, give 15 drops of tincture three times a day. The tea and tincture are bitter and may need to be sweetened with honey for children.

FROM THE AUTHOR'S JOURNAL
AUGUST 18

I wake up full of craziness left over from yesterday. Too many things to do, too many necessary chores crunched into one small day, and too many things lined up already for today. Who can do so many things and still stay close to sane? To calm myself, I grab a basket to work on and sit outside on the dooryard steps.

The morning sounds like fall. A cool wind blows and blows, and leaves rustle, and long grasses in the field shush and flatten. There are clouds, and a sprinkle of leftover rain drips from the roof. Water stands like beaded silver on the iris leaves, and on the grass, and in the angled joints of sunflower stems. At the steps where I sit, the chipmunk darts out and scares me. He races up the steps after breakfast seed. I thought he was a leaf until he ran over my feet, and I screech, and he runs off to sit quivering under the steps, hoping for me to go inside.

In the garden, there are tomatoes that scream to be picked. I put down the basket, grab a pot, and bring lots of bright red fruit into the kitchen. The ripest tomatoes get chopped up along with onions and garlic and herbs for a sauce, and everything gets set on the stove to simmer.

On the table lies the blue vervain I brought in last night and was too tired to process. A week or so ago, I saw it growing down by Stevens Brook, along the rocky, rubbly soil that banks the water. It grew beside a few scraggly dock plants already gone to seed, a huge barberry, and a few boneset plants, all eking out a life from the deep underground water beneath the poor-looking soil. That was the first time I've seen it here, although I've used it elsewhere to help calm nerves. I decide that maybe it would help me now, and fix a cup of hot tea with some of the leaves and flowers.

While the tea cools, I leaf through herb books and stir the tomato sauce, sipping at the hot vervain tea. It is bitter, but not terrible, and I finish the whole cup soon. After half and hour or so, I feel better. Maybe it was the vervain, or maybe it was just sitting still for a while. In any case, I'm grateful for vervain, and ready for another day.

Kitchen Notes

I gather up the plants brought in earlier, and decide to use some for tincture. They get chopped up and put in a jar with alcohol. Some of the tiny dark purple blossoms fall off and I rescue them for the tincture jar. The rest of the plants I bundle to dry, now that I know that the taste is not too awful. Even hanging upside down from the drying rack, they still look impressive, stiff and formal, with little bits of purple flower fluff at their tips.

Experiences with Vervain

I've used vervain before, in tincture form, mostly for nervousness and anxiety, and especially for the kids when they were sick and cranky and restless. A few drops of the tincture mixed up in a spoonful of honey helped them rest, making recovery a little easier for all of us.

COLTSFOOT
Tussilago farfara

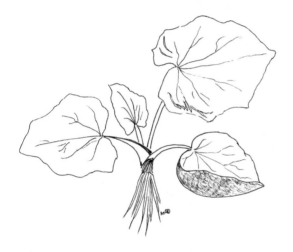

Reflections: Everything rustles in a wind that has blown all day. Sumac leaves shift and flutter, and the long grasses flatten and sway. I kneel to pick coltsfoot for tea. Poking through the thick and fuzzy leaves, I surprise the chipmunk and he cheeps at me in alarm, and darts away. I chew on a coltsfoot leaf, and wonder if the chipmunk eats them, too, as a tasty green addition to his diet.

Description: Coltsfoot is a low-growing perennial plant found in moist waste places, on streambanks, and along damp roadsides. In the wild, coltsfoot can occur in huge mats, and it is sometimes planted in shady area as a ground cover.

Coltsfoot's leaves appear as the flowers are dying back. They are basal, between 2 and 7 inches long, and often as wide. The leaves are roughly heart-shaped, supposedly resembling the outline of a colt's hoofprint. Leaf margins are unevenly toothed and shallowly lobed. Leaves are pale grayish green on the surface. Underneath, they are covered with a whitish downy fluff. Plant height can be up to 18 inches high.

The flowers arrive in very early spring, before the leaves appear, and look a bit like dandelion blossoms. The plant is a Composite family member, with flowers having a central disk surrounded by bright yellow ray flowers. The flower head is up to 1 inch wide, and blossoms occur atop single stalks that sprout from creeping underground runners. The stalk is leafless, having small bracts along its length. Blossoms occur in very early spring, and then fade back to produce fluffy seed heads like dandelions.

Medicinal Uses: Coltsfoot is known primarily for its effect on the respiratory system. It is expectorant, demulcent, and antispasmodic. The leaves, flowers, and root will act to soothe inflamed respiratory membranes, aiding in the expectoration of mucus and helping to calm a cough. These actions make it a useful remedy in asthma or bronchitis, as well as in common coughs or colds. It can also be used in chronic emphysema to help soothe irritated membranes. Coltsfoot's demulcent action makes it useful in treating sore throats. Native Americans smoked the dried plant for asthma, bronchitis, and whooping cough. The dried plant was used traditionally as a base for cough drops or lozenges.

Coltsfoot is also diuretic, and it can be used in mild bladder inflammations where it will help ease the passage of urine and soothe inflamed membranes. Externally, coltsfoot is emollient, working to soothe skin on contact, and the fresh, crushed leaves can be used as a poultice to help in healing damaged skin.

Harvesting: The blossoms may be picked in very early spring, just as they are opening. Leaves can be gathered throughout the growing season, early spring through fall, as long as they look healthy and green. The whole plant can be pulled up and processed immediately to make a fresh-plant tincture. Or the leaves and flowers and root can be dried, and used later as a tea. The leaves are somewhat fleshy, so should be spread on screens or baskets, and turned often to ensure proper air exposure.

Dosages: For coltsfoot tea, use one tablespoon of dried herb to 1 cup of boiling water, steep 10–20 minutes, and drink hot three times daily. The tincture is used in doses of 30–40 drops three times daily. For skin wounds and irritations, crush the fresh leaf and apply to the cleansed area as a poultice.

CAUTION: Coltsfoot contains potentially toxic alkaloids that can be harmful if taken in large doses over long periods of time. Do not exceed recommended dosages. Coltsfoot should not be taken by pregnant or nursing women.

FROM THE AUTHOR'S JOURNAL
AUGUST 20

A nice day. There is a cloud covering the sun for just a moment, and a little chill makes me put on a flannel shirt. The breeze rustles leaves of the tall sunflowers near the steps. All day long, birds have fluttered at the feeder, scrounging for the little seed that is left. And the hummingbirds have droned past my head on their way to the red sugar water hung from the sumacs. The air is dry and nice.

On the dooryard porch, fat braids of onions sit in the sun to cure. And on the ground, more lay out to dry a bit before they get stored. Bees sit in the sunflower disks. I wish the sunflowers could last forever, but then, of course, they wouldn't make the seeds the birds love. Yesterday the chipmunk climbed up a thick stalk and sat comfortably on the nodded neck of the tallest sunflower. What a wonderful thing, to sit on a sunflower! I watched him at the kitchen door while he groomed himself and watched me watching him.

The sky is full of patchy clouds. In the back field, reddish seckle pears blush, not quite ready yet. This morning I walked out to look at them. Already winds have forced some of them to the ground, and the fallen ones are marked with the teeth of the deer who come at night. I tasted a couple and the flavor is good, but they are still hard and puckery.

So many things are ripe these days I could harvest all day long and still not have enough time. Down the road, blackberries are fat and dark and juicy. Every morning's walk feeds me. And in the garden, tomatoes happen so fast we don't have enough places to put them. The hyssop is starting to bloom, and the echinacea is full of perfect, bristly green buds. Under the sumacs, where the violets bloomed and then stopped, now thistles and giant violet leaves crowd, covering the coltsfoot.

I missed coltsfoot in the spring. Every year, I forget to watch for its flower, which comes just as the snow melts away. Now I squat to find the leaves that are hidden under the jungly growth. Pushing back tall heart-shaped leaves of the violets and gently moving the prickly thistles aside, I search along the ground and find the first of tiny leaves that creeps through the grass. These baby leaves come first, like scouts, to widen the coltsfoot's territory. One tiny leaf leads to another larger leaf, and then to the clump of coltsfoot tucked around a huge rock that borders one side of the garden.

I pluck one of the larger leaves. It is green on the surface and fuzzy and whitish underneath. I take a bite, and it is thick and tasty. My sister says that Native Americans wrapped food in coltsfoot for cooking, to season it, but I haven't tried that yet.

Several years ago, I found three coltsfoot plants here in the damp and shaded soil. They spread now, a few inches at a time, keeping us supplied with enough leaves for tea each year. I gather some of the larger leaves now, plopping them in my shirttail, holding it up like an apron, and go inside to spread them out to dry.

Experiences with Coltsfoot

My daughter has used coltsfoot in an asthma tea for years, and found it helpful, and we've depended on it for gentle help with coughs. Last year I tried making coltsfoot cough drops with maple syrup instead of sugar, but they didn't turn out right. They never quite got hard. My daughter said they tasted great, though, and took the sticky powdery blobs to school where she and her friend ate them like candy. Neither of the girls coughed after that, but they weren't sick so it's not a fair test. Maybe I'll try again this year, and use sugar instead.

BLACKBERRY
Rubus allegheniensis and species

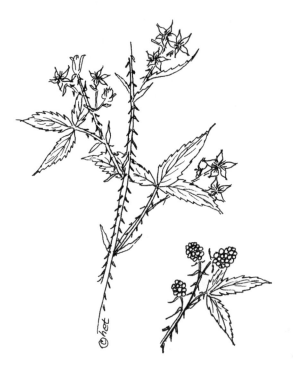

Reflections: There are no sounds in the woods this morning, except the dripping of last night's rain from one leaf to another. When I reach the clearing where the blackberries grow, rain starts again, so hard that I take shelter under a canopy of beech and hemlock. It pours for a long while—long enough for me to stand still and close my eyes and sink my own roots deep into the woodland soil.

Description: Of the numerous blackberry species in the Northeast, the one most likely to be found is the common blackberry, *Rubus allegheniensis*. It is a prickly-stemmed plant and is a member of the Rose family, as attested to by its thorns. All blackberry species may be found in dry thickets and clearings where they form thick thorny hedges. Blackberry is often one of the first plants to reclaim disturbed soil.

The leaves are alternate and divided into 3 or 5 sharply toothed leaflets. Small, sharp thorns grow on the undersurface of leaves as well as along the stems. Plant height may be up to 8 feet.

The flowers are white with five petals; blossoms about 1 inch wide, and petals are longer than sepals. Common blackberry flowers occur in racemes, in spring and summer, but other species bloom from spring through fall.

The fruit is a shiny, juicy, black berry containing seeds; it is sweet in some species, astringent in others, and is edible. Fruit of the common blackberry can be used interchangeably for medicinal purposes.

Medicinal Uses: Blackberry's primary medicinal property is its sharp and strong astringency. The leaves, fruit, and root bark can be used. The astringency makes blackberry a useful remedy for simple diarrhea, where it will help reduce inflammation and tone irritated membranes. It can be used, too, in dysentery, where its hemostatic properties as well as its astringency will help stop bloody diarrhea.

Blackberry's astringency makes it useful, also, as a gargle for sore throats when there is redness and swelling. Used as a mouthwash several times a day, it can be helpful for mouth sores or ulcers, too.

Harvesting: The fruit can be gathered when it is fully ripe and then dried to use later as a tea. Berries should be spread one layer thick on a screen, or they can be spread on a cookie sheet and dried slowly at very low temperatures in the oven. To make a syrup, the juice can be expressed from fresh berries and simmered with honey over a low heat. Leaves can be harvested any time when they are green and healthy looking. Spread these out to dry, taking care to avoid thorns, and store when fully dry for use later. The root can be gathered either before flowers appear or after green material has died back in late fall. Cut the roots from the plant, rinse well, and peel the root bark away. Cut the root bark into this strips and spread to dry on screens. Store when thoroughly dry.

Dosages: Use 1–2 tablespoons of the dried leaves or root to 1 cup of boiling water for tea, and drink three times daily. If using the root bark, place 1–2 teaspoons of dried bark into 2 cups of water, and simmer on low heat for about 10 minutes. Use ¹/₂ cup of this mixture three or four times daily. Syrup can be taken three times daily, using ¹/₂–1 teaspoon per dose.

FROM THE AUTHOR'S JOURNAL
AUGUST 21

Near the clearing where blackberries grow, light filters in and I stand at the wood's edge, sniffing and looking around. Deer and other animals must come here, and I am still for a moment to check for any signs of them. Then I step out of the woods.

Tall ferns stand everywhere, like green frilly fans, and woven over and around them are tough blackberry vines. The stems are red and full of nasty thorns that grab at me when I pass them. Every step I take toward the berries is careful. I pluck my shirttail or sleeve away and hold my arms close.

There are lots of berries, ripe and black, and I start picking, putting them in a bag I brought and eating a few as I go. A little breeze starts up. The berries I reach for dance out of my hand, and I have to hold the vine to keep it still. The more berries I pick, the more I see. The fattest, juiciest ones are one more step into the brambles, one more step away.

Some of the vines are new shoots, with fine, soft green leaves and no berries, and I decide to gather blackberry leaves to use for tea. The leaves are prickly underneath, and gathering them is sticky business. I hold each leaf tip carefully, and tear it away from its stem. The wind picks up, and rain starts again, but I keep picking anyway, calmed and refreshed. When the rain slows to a sprinkle again and my bag is full, I walk down the hill to the road.

Kitchen Notes

By the time I get home, my hair is damp curls and my feet are numb with cold. I dump blackberries out into a bowl on the table, and arrange leaves on baskets to dry. Water gets heated for blackberry leaf tea, and I pull on dry socks. I taste a plump, glossy berry that is sweet and full of flavor. I eat another, and another, until half of them are gone. Maybe next time I gather blackberries I'll make a syrup of them to use for diarrhea. The root bark is strongly astringent; when simmered in a syrup of the berries, it makes a strong medicine for diarrhea. It would be fun to make my own syrup, if I can figure out how to dig up blackberry roots without getting scratched to death. In the meantime, I've got leaves drying and fruit to eat. I'll think about roots later.

JEWELWEED
Impatiens capensis and *pallida*

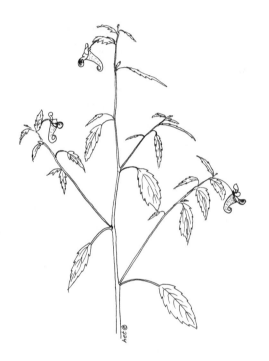

Reflections: It's a wonderful day. The air is cold, about 42 degrees, and the grass is still wet with drops of dew that dampen my feet. The sky is clear and blue. Sun coming up brightens the sunflowers and makes glittery spots on all the damp leaves. I put jewelweed samples in the plant press where the blossoms are a shock of orange against the ivory page.

Description: A tall, pretty plant of wet woods and shady meadows and along streambanks, jewelweed is commonly known as touch-me-not. Two species of jewelweed can be used medicinally, and they are used interchangeably. In both species, the flower is oddly shaped and very attractive, and some jewelweeds are planted as ornamentals.

Jewelweed leaves occur along a pale green stem. They are softly toothed, and they repel water. The plant is called jewelweed because drops of rain or dew bead up like crystal droplets on the leaf surfaces, which never seem to get wet. The leaves grow up to 3 inches in length, with pale undersides. Leaves are oval or egg shaped. Plant height can be up to 6 feet.

In the spotted touch-me-not, *Impatiens capensis,* blossoms are true orange, with reddish brown spots. The flower has a sharply curved spur at the rear.

In the pale touch-me-not, *Impatiens pallida,* the blossom is similar in shape, but is bright to pale yellow, with only a few pale brownish spots in its throat. This blossom gets a bit larger, up to 1 1/2 inches long, and is about as wide as it is long. The rear spur is somewhat shorter than *Impatiens capensis.* In both species, flowers occur form early summer through fall.

Both jewelweeds bear a fruit that is a swollen-appearing capsule that explodes with an audible sound when touched, hence its common name of touch-me-not. The capsule splits into two tight spirals, and the seed is flung about over the nearby ground.

Medicinal Uses: Jewelweed had a fairly specific and limited medicinal use, but it is effective and good to know about in survival situations. The freshly crushed plant helps control the itching of skin irritations, and it is a specific traditional remedy for poison ivy. If rubbed over the skin, or used as a strong wash soon after exposure to poison ivy, jewelweed can help prevent development or worsening of the allergic reaction. A poultice or strong wash or both can also heal a rash that has already developed. Jewelweed is also fungicidal, and it can be used on athlete's foot with good relief.

Harvesting: The whole aboveground plant is used. Gather the fresh plant any time it is flowering. To use in the wild, simply crush and apply to the affected area. At home, you can pour a small amount of boiling water over the fresh plant soon after gathering, let it steep for half an hour, and apply the liquid as a wash several times a day. If you will not be using the plant immediately, wild foods naturalist Euell Gibbons suggests pureeing it in a blender with a little water, and freezing the mixture in ice-cube trays to use later. Jewelweed can also be tinctured, and the tincture used externally.

Dosages: The fresh plant is crushed and applied to affected skin as a poultice, and changed several times daily. Or a strong tea can be made and poured over cloth that is applied directly to the skin and held in place with gauze. If large areas of skin are affected, use a large container to make a very strong tea to pour into a bathtub. Soak for 15–20 minutes several times a day in the jewelweed bathwater.

FROM THE AUTHOR'S JOURNAL
AUGUST 23

This morning mist spreads like a blanket around the mountains and over the lake. I am out when only a thin strip of orange shows at the horizon, and walk in the mostly dark. At Weeks's farm the cows are a cluster of dots near the woods, huddled together for warmth.

Down the development road, if the fox I saw yesterday is watching me, I don't notice, but he can easily hide in the shadowy half-light. I watch for mint and boneset and bugleweed, checking their progress. They are all still blooming and look fine.

At the swampy place where the stream still flows, turtlehead stands in the middle of water and mucky earth, and I decide to take some home if I can get it. The earth that used to be woodland is soft and full of the fiber of rotting trees, and I sink into it, but my feet stay dry. Near the water, I step on roots and fallen limbs and make my way carefully to the turtlehead. But not close enough. Just one, long, impossible step away, it stands in flower.

I sit on a stump and look around. The air is clear and cold. My breath is frosty and puffs away in little clouds. I decide to leave the turtlehead. If it's this hard to get to, it must not be right for me to pick it.

Up the road toward home, where the stream still trickles and keeps the soil wet, sedges grow bright, light green. Jewelweed stands in bloom, full of odd-shaped, speckled blossoms that dangle and dance in the breeze. I pick some to put in the plant press, and look around for jewelweed's common neighbor, poison ivy. Close by, the telltale stubble from last year still holds white berries. These two plants often grow near each other—a handy arrangement, since jewelweed is a remedy for poison ivy reaction. I don't usually react to poison ivy, but lots of people do. I decide to gather a bunch of jewelweed to have around in case someone needs it, and break off a few of the pretty plants to take home. The stalks snap off easily and lots of juice leaks from the broken end. Two sprigs with perfect flowers will go into the plant press at home.

Back over the rougher and dryer ground, I climb through blackberry brambles. The berries are fat and long and cold in the cool morning air, and wet with dew. I eat as I walk, and decide to come here later to pick more. But not too many. All the animals here depend on them for food, and for me it's just a treat. Clutching the sparkly jewelweed, I make my way home as sun creeps from behind a shroud of mist.

WILD LETTUCE
Lactuca species

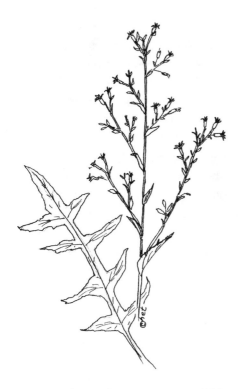

Reflections: Next to the wild lettuce, a field looks like magic. It is covered with soft glittery purple fur. On closer inspection, the fur turns out to be fluffy-topped grasses with tiny red flowers, all weighted down with the silvery rain. I pick a wet sprig to look up at home, and tuck it into my pack with the wild lettuce that still holds raindrops beaded on its blue-green leaves.

Description: Several species of *Lactuca* occur in the Northeast and can be used interchangeably. Two of the most commonly used varieties are wild lettuce, *Lactuca canadensis,* and prickly lettuce, *Lactuca scariola.* The leaves and stems of all species release a milky juice when torn or crushed.

Wild lettuce frequents fields, clearings, and disturbed soil, and it can also be found bordering woodlands. Its leaves vary from deeply lobed to smooth edged, and may be up to 1 foot long. The leaves occur alternately and are often toothed. This species may attain 10 feet in height. The flower heads are pale yellow, about ¼ inch wide, and occur in long clusters. Plants can be seen in bloom in summer and fall.

The fruit consists of tiny seeds attached to bristly hairs that carry the seed through the air.

Prickly lettuce is commonly found in waste places and along roadsides. The leaves of this species are up to 1 foot long and may be lobed or not. They are oblong in shape, and the leaf margins are very prickly. A line of bristles also runs along the midvein underneath the leaves. Leaves clasp the stem at their bases. Plant height is up to 5 feet. The flowers are yellow and about $1/4$ inch wide. The blossoms are yellow ray flowers that occur summer through fall. Flowers soon give way to seeds that are carried by bristly hairs attached to the seed.

Medicinal Uses: All species, including the common garden lettuce to some extent, have mild sedative properties. The *Lactucas* may be used to help relieve nervousness and irritability and in some cases may be helpful in relieving insomnia. This herb is especially useful for children when they are sick and irritable and have trouble resting enough to recuperate. *Lactuca* is bitter, though, and will probably need to be sweetened with honey for taste when given to children.

Lactuca has also been noted as an anodyne and used to relieve mild pain. It can be helpful in arthritis or rheumatism, and in menstrual cramps, it can be added to other herbs for pain relief.

In general, the wild lettuces are gentle in action and can be helpful whenever a mild sedative, tranquilizing action is desired.

Harvesting: Gather the leaves of *Lactuca* species in summer when they are healthy and lush, and especially when they are flowering. Dry leaves by spreading on screens or baskets, and keep out of the sun. Turn every other day or so until dry. Cut and store when ready. A fresh-plant tincture can be made of the leaves upon gathering, or a dried-plant tincture can be prepared later.

Dosages: For a tea, make an infusion using 1–2 tablespoons of dried leaves to 1 cup of boiling water, and steep for 20 minutes. Drink two or three times daily. If giving to children, mix in some honey or other natural sweetener to improve taste, and give in $1/4$–$1/2$ cup doses three times daily. The tincture may be given three times daily in doses of 30 drops for adults and 5–15 drops for children, depending on age and size.

The air outside has just an edge of chill, and the wet grass is cold to walk in. Last night for the third time in a row, rain poured on and off. This early morning, clouds still covered the sky but now blue is showing through. A fan of sun lights up the goldfinches at the feeder and the wet sumac trees.

As I walk along the road, I notice the usual litter of dead frogs. Last night, driving home in the rain, lots of them sailed across the road, lit gold by the glow of my headlights. They plopped quickly along the wet road, but it's hard to avoid them all. I wonder why they come out so in the rain? Maybe water builds up in the ditches and flushes them from their homes. Or maybe little pools and wet spots fill, and they travel to mate or lay eggs. In any case, there are more of them on the road to-day. Even in the still-dark, I can see them lying in weird shapes, with slugs gathered around to feed on the soft remains.

Porter Road is still full of shadows when I start down, and in the si-lence my footsteps are loud, one gravelly crunch after another. I am sure there are animals nearby, being still until I pass, but I don't see them. When the light comes a bit, the vegetation shows lush and per-fect along the narrow roadbanks, and I walk a long, green, and wet tunnel.

Where a path enters the dirt road toward home, wild lettuce stands tall—a single plant here and there, flowers in full bloom. The flowers that have gone by are yellowish and scraggly looking. Fluffs of seed make some plants look bedraggled, but the pointy, divided leaves are still pretty, and when I pluck one, white latex beads up at the torn edge. I pick one giant plant to take home. Its main stem has been broken off, and several side shoots are tall and full of buds. Soon, my hands feel sticky and I glance down to see they are full of milky sap.

There are not so many plants here along the edges of the woods as I see in other places. In the city, wild lettuce sprouts in every rubbly lot, from cracks in the sidewalk to the bases of building foundations. Here, they seem to be scarcer, so I take just a few of the plants. I chew a bit of leaf but spit it out soon. It reminds me of the lettuce in the garden when it starts to bolt—strong flavored and bitter tasting. I make my way with the prickly plants through a damp field and home.

Kitchen Notes

Two years ago I made a wild lettuce tincture that has lasted until now. Today's herb will go for a new batch. I chop the prickly leaves into small bits. The milky juice flows, gumming up the scissors and making my fingers sticky. Alcohol poured over the pieces turns cloudy and then green. After a while, the latex on my fingers wears away, but the bitterness persists, and I know I'll have to serve this herb in honey to hide the taste.

Experiences with Wild Lettuce

I've used wild lettuce in a tincture for the kids when they were sick and cranky. It helped make staying in bed easier for them, and it made sick-time easier for all of us.

WILD CHERRY
Prunus serotina and species

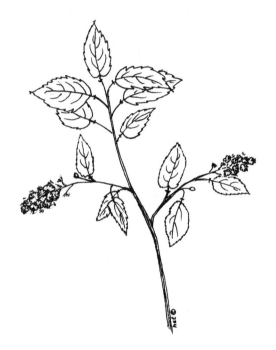

Reflections: All the trees are tinged with scarlet now, and the bright leaves ripple in a little breeze. The bark that slips away from the tiny cherry tree smells so intense it makes my mouth water, and I tear off a little piece to chew. The young bull watching me must like the scent, too. He bobs closer and noses at the pocket that holds the purple strips. I offer him a bit and he snuffs at it for a second, then pokes out a huge, pale tongue. We stand in the amber field under a flawless sky, chewing cherry bark together.

Description: The official wild cherry of herbal tradition is the black cherry, *Prunus serotina*. Other cherry species may be used medicinally for the same purposes, although the chokecherry, *Prunus virginiana*, should be avoided since its bark can be toxic. The wild black cherry tree may attain 80 feet in height, with foliage and bark that have a distinct, aromatic, cherry odor. The tree is common throughout the Northeast and grows in a variety of soils and regions as well.

The leaves are oblong or elliptical in shape. They are up to 5 inches long, and the margins are bluntly toothed. Each leaf has a pair of dark red glands at the base. The leaves are dark green and glossy on the surface and lighter underneath. When the leaves are crushed, a strong aromatic scent of cherry is released.

Wild black cherry flowers are about ¹/₂ inch wide, with five rounded white petals. Blossoms occur in racemes that are 4 to 6 inches long, and these spring from the leaf axils. The tree flowers spring to early summer.

Fruit is a dark reddish-black cherry with a central stone. It occurs along the stem projecting from leaf axils and is edible although somewhat bitter. The cherries ripen in late summer and are about ¹/₂ inch in diameter.

Medicinal Uses: The bark of the wild cherry is expectorant, antispasmodic, and antitussive. These properties indicate its usefulness as a preparation for coughs, where it will inhibit the cough reflex and ease spasmodic coughing. A syrup of wild cherry is often used as a base for commercial cough medicines for this reason. Wild cherry is best employed when coughing is spasmodic and relentless, making resting at night difficult. Wild cherry can be added to preparations for bronchitis or whooping cough and can be helpful in coughs that accompany pneumonia. It is also helpful in coughs with influenza, where there is associated shortness of breath.

Harvesting: The inner bark may be gathered from the tree in fall after the fruit has matured. Using a drawknife, or other sharp knife, slice into the outer bark and peel it away in strips. The inner bark will be greenish white in color and can be separated from the reddish grey outer bark. Be careful not to remove the bark from the tree in a complete circle and thus kill the tree. Spread out the bark strips to dry along screens, baskets, or paper bags, and keep out of the sun. When brittle enough to snap easily, store for later use in tightly closed containers.

Dosages: For tea, make a decoction with 1 tablespoon of dried inner bark to 1 cup of boiling water. Simmer 15–20 minutes, strain, and drink the tea three times daily. A tincture may be made of the dried or fresh bark and used in place of the tea. The tincture should be taken in 15–20 drop doses three times a day. A cold infusion may be made from wild cherry bark, by placing 1 ounce of the dried bark into 1 pint of cool water and allowing to sit overnight of for 6–8 hours. Strain out the bark, and drink in $^1/_2$–1 cup doses three times a day.

Wild cherry can also be used in syrup form by covering the dried inner bark with an equal volume in honey, and simmering the mixture over very low heat for 30–60 minutes, or in a Crock–Pot on low setting overnight. Strain out plant material, and give $^1/_4$ to $^1/_2$ teaspoon of the resulting syrup three times a day.

CAUTION: Since wild cherry acts to suppress a cough, it should not be used in large doses. A cough is a natural process that breaks up congestion and removes it from the body.

FROM THE AUTHOR'S JOURNAL
AUGUST 31

Outside in the yard, sun that has stolen over the horizon paints the grass golden and glistens on dewdrops. The light is mellow, full of magic, and everything glows in it. Long shadows of cosmos and snapdragons stretch across the lawn, quivering in a faint breeze. Yesterday the lawn was mowed, and today it looks neat and even—a surprise after so many days of bushy carpet. Now the plantain and shepherd's purse and clover are all tucked into green anonymity again. Today I am out to check for wild cherry bark. It's still early in the season but lately the air is cool and dry, and a few scarlet patches have started in the summer-green trees. I pack the drawknife and set off for Big Sandy. The best trees are in a small clump on Porter Road, but this morning I'm late and there isn't enough time to go that far. At a neighboring farm, there are young cherry trees that line the edges of a field, so I'll check them.

By the time I get to the farm, the air is well lit already, and the cows stand under the apple trees. One walks slowly, grazing, while her calf nurses from behind, struggling to keep up. They stare at me and are quiet when I pass. A young bull walks closer, his huge head bobbing as his body sways toward me, following my progress. I stop at a little cherry sapling, and check the leaf glands for color. These little bumpy projections on either side of the stem at the leaf base should be red on the black cherry, *Prunus serotina*—the official medicinal tree. Most of the cherries have the same properties, but I figure there must be a reason why this particular species was chosen, so I look for it. The leaf glands on this cherry are dark red. Its bark is smooth, almost silky, maroon in color, with light speckles throughout. There are no branches extending from it yet, just one narrow trunk—a young tree.

I place the drawknife high in the air against the trunk and pull downward; a thin strip of purply bark curls toward me. Underneath, the wood is pale. The bark that peels away is shiny and dark, and smells intensely of cherry. I pop a bit of it in my mouth and chew for a minute. It is astringent, and a little bitter. I expected the bark to taste fruity, but it doesn't, at least not so far. I gather more while the cows watch, and fill a pocket. The tree where I work is small, and soon I have gathered all the bark that is safe for this tree to give up, and all I have time for today. The bark fills one pocket, enough for a few cups of tea or a tiny tincture, or maybe to cook down as a syrup. In another month or so when the frosts come, I'll try the trees down Porter Road. There the cherries are ripening already and are sweet enough to eat right from the tree. The bark should be good, too. Walking home, I fill my other pocket with blackberries and bid the cows good-bye.

Kitchen Notes

In the kitchen, I pull little scraps of bark out of my pockets and spread the smaller bits along a screen. Some are starting to dry already, and curl up at either end, but are still pliable. I peel off the rough outer bark of the big pieces and spread the pale inner bark out to dry next to the first batch. The work is a little tedious, for the bark is thin. By the time I've completed my task, the deep and fragrant scent of cherry fills the house.

Experiences with Wild Cherry

Several years ago , I had a persistent chest cold and couldn't finish a sentence without coughing long and hard. Small amounts of wild cherry bark in a cough syrup made a real difference in just one day. I put wild cherry, too, in a cough formula for a friend who couldn't sleep through the night due to coughing. Even a small dose helped, allowing her to get much-needed rest.

JUNIPER
Juniperus species

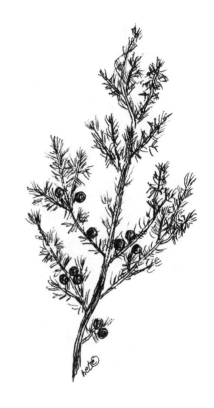

Reflections: On the way back down the path I lie on soft needles for a while. The earth smells wonderful, close and peaceful, and full of magic. The scents are intense and curious—the clear and calming smell of balsam, a deep, woodsy fragrance of earth and mushrooms rotting, all broken by the sweet, musky scent of an animal nearby. I brush pine needles from my hair and smell juniper. Holding my pocket full of berries, I get up and move on down the hill.

Description: Various juniper species grow in the Northeast and all have the same medicinal uses. The most widespread species in the region is Eastern red cedar, *Juniperus virginiana,* which is seen as an evergreen tree up to 60 feet in height, but common juniper, *Juniperus communis,* is the juniper of herbal tradition. It is most often a short shrub that grows in clumps along rocky forest areas or in fields. It is sometimes seen as a small, spreading tree, but generally will only attain 4 feet in height and more often is seen at 1 to 2 foot levels.

The bark of the shrub or tree is scaly and generally reddish or gray in color. It is often seen hanging in shreds from branches.

The leaves of common juniper occur as evergreen needles that are up to ¹/₂ inch in length and are very sharply pointed. They are stiff, and are bluish green in color with a whitish cast to them. The needles grow along the stem at right angles and are uncomfortable to touch. When crushed, the needles emit a strong aromatic scent.

Fruit of *Juniperus communis* is a berrylike cone that is ¹/₄ to ¹/₂ inch in diameter. It is dusky blue with a white cast to it that can be wiped off with the fingers. (The white coating, called a "bloom," is a naturally occurring yeast that is found on some wild fruits, including blueberries.) The juniper berry is hard and mealy in texture and somewhat oily. It can be found on the bushes first as a green berry that ripens to its typical blue color. The berries, when crushed, release an intensely aromatic odor. Each fruit of common juniper contains one to three seeds, and the berries remain attached to the branch until eaten by wildlife.

Medicinal Uses: The dried, mature juniper berries are diuretic and antiseptic. They can be used to treat mild bladder infections or irritations, where they will increase urine output and help reduce bacteria populations. Juniper berries should not, however, be used where there is chronic kidney infection, since the oils are too stimulating and may be irritating to the kidneys. Juniper berries are also carminative and can be taken before a meal, at which time they will stimulate the digestive juices of the stomach and aid in digestion. The berries are often used in preparing wild meats, enhancing the flavor and supporting digestion.

Externally, a poultice of the crushed berries can be applied to inflamed joint areas in rheumatism or arthritis.

Harvesting: Gather the individual berries when they are dark blue to purple. Dry by spreading out on screens or other appropriate material. Store after 2 weeks or when all moisture has been removed.

Dosages: Place 1 tablespoon of dried, crushed berries in a cup, and pour boiling water over them. Allow the tea to steep for 20–30 minutes, and remove the plant material. The infusion can be drunk three times daily.

To use externally for joint inflammations, pour a bit of boiling water over the dried berries, let sit for 5 minutes, then pour off water and crush berries. Apply them to a clean cloth, and place over the affected area. Repeat several times a day.

CAUTION: Juniper berries should be avoided during pregnancy, as the oils may affect tissues of the uterus. Juniper should also be avoided in active or chronic kidney disease, as the oils are too irritating and stimulating in those cases.

FROM THE AUTHOR'S JOURNAL
SEPTEMBER 4

This morning, a Sunday, there is time for a leisurely walk, and I decide to try the road that splits off from Big Sandy and winds up through the woods. Thick growth in these woods and a lack of time have kept me away, but today is quiet, and I've got some extra time.

The sky is a sheet of gray outside, and over the mountains an unbroken rope of cloud hovers. A chill in the air makes me a little sad at the passing of summer. Down Big Sandy nothing stirs. There are two tiny shrews dead in the road, soft and furry, and I pick them up by the tail and put them in the grass. Alongside the road, wintergreen grows thick and I sit to pick a handful of new dark leaves to dry for tea. I lean over to see a ground bird patrolling an area hidden by low hemlock branches. He scuffles to and fro in the pine litter and makes funny, garbly sounds as he goes. From what I can see, it is a mottled-brownish color, and I guess that it is a grouse. When I shift positions, the bird flaps off in a burst of sound, and I get up and keep on walking.

The path splits off into the woods, and I follow it to cross a section of grasses, sedges, and self-heal. The ground is damp and dark and packed down firm, and the walking is hard. The earth is ridged and broken by so many tracks that my ankles twist if I walk too fast. Deer and moose (and maybe even bear) travel this road.

Soon the soil is drier, and juniper takes over a ridge of earth. It stands in big, bristly clumps reaching far up along the hill. I check among the bluish needles and find berries studding the rough-barked branches. Some of them are already turning blue. They are all covered with the white "bloom" that is a naturally occurring yeast. It rubs off when I roll the berry between my fingers. When the yeast is gone, a pattern of white lines like a starburst shows at the bottom. I take one firm berry and split it open with a thumbnail. Inside the hard fruit, there are three seeds lined up and buried in greenish brown flesh.

I start picking the ripe fruit, but it's not easy. The juniper needles stick out every which way and stab at me. I suffer through a few branches and pick a handful of berries to get a head start on the season. Close by, two loons cry to each other again and again. Beyond my eye's reach, they dart back and forth with their lilting, haunting cry. They seem to ask a question, plaintive. I stand to listen for a while, hoping they'll cross this clearing. They stay hidden, though, and after a while, I take my juniper home.

Experiences with Juniper

For years now, I've used juniper in tea form for bladder infections. Usually I add it to other herbs, such as pipsissewa, horsetail, or cleavers, and the berries give the tea a wonderful scent, as well as providing good medicine.

Hops
Humulus lupulus

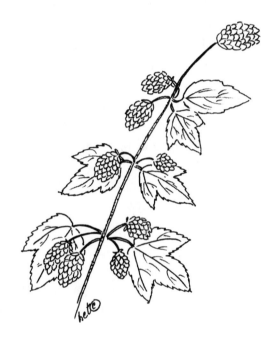

Reflections: It's such an exciting time, these harvesting days. Everything is fruiting, racing to set its seed as the air gets colder and the first light frosts chill the nights. Yesterday I found hops, full of fluffy apple-green seed heads. Such pretty flowery things, they ran along a vine up and over some rocks. Somehow it seems right that something so beautiful should be so useful, too.

Description: Hops is found in the wild as a vine within rich thickets and moist forest areas. The plant can often be found in dense mats, or it can be seen in trees that it climbs and uses for support. Leaves are up to 5 inches in length and width and have a coarse surface. They have 3 to 5 sharply pointed lobes, with roughly toothed margins, and somewhat resemble grape leaves. The leaves occur along the woody stem; stems may be up to 30 or 40 feet in length, although they often twine together, thus appearing shorter.

Flowers appear in the plant in mid- to late summer. Male and female blossoms occur on different plants. The male flowers are small and inconspicuous, with five petals. They occur in loose bunches.

Female flowers are inconspicuous and occur in pairs, later maturing into fruit.

The fruit, or strobile, is a drooping, conelike cluster of overlapping bracts. This strobile is pale green in color until it ripens in the fall, when it turns pale amber and becomes covered with a yellow powder. The strobile of hops is the part used medicinally.

Medicinal Uses: Hops has several properties that make it a useful remedy for in nervous disorders or digestive complaints. The strobiles are sedative and calming and help to relieve pain. They are useful in insomnia, muscle tension, and general restlessness. The herb is also a bitter tonic and will help relieve indigestion and nervous stomach in tense situations. Hops are also astringent and antiseptic and can be helpful is colitis, where it will not only help tone tissues and reduce inflammation, but also aid in relaxation.

Externally, the strobiles can be used as a poultice that will have an antibiotic effect on skin ulcers or abcesses or poorly healing sores. Hops has also been used to stuff "dream pillows" used to treat insomnia where the strong aromatic scent is said to induce sleep.

Harvesting: The strobiles are the part used. Gather the vine when strobiles are turning from pale green to yellowish brown and are covered with a yellow powder. The strobiles can be dried on their vines if drying conditions are excellent—that is, hot and very dry days. If the weather is humid or cloudy, it is best to remove strobiles and dry them one layer thick on a cookie sheet in the oven. Set temperature at its lowest reading, and prop the oven door open to allow moisture to escape. Whether air dried or oven dried, as soon as strobiles are crumbly to the touch, store immediately in airtight containers. Hops will spoil easily if not completely dry. Hops loses its potency after about 6 months, so it is best to tincture whatever you won't be using within that time period.

Dosages: For tea, use 1 heaping tablespoon of dried strobiles to 1 cup of boiling water. Steep 15–30 minutes, and drink several times daily, or just before bedtime if used for insomnia. If using tincture, take 20–40 drops three or four times daily or before bedtime.

To use externally, crush hops and moisten with hot water or cider vinegar. Apply to the affected skin, and cover with a hot, moist towel. Repeat several times a day.

CAUTION: Hops should not be used internally where there is chronic depression, as it can exacerbate that condition.

FROM THE AUTHOR'S JOURNAL
SEPTEMBER 13

I am going away for a week, and have mixed feelings about it. I know it will be good to get away, and to see plants that grow in another place, but it's hard to tear myself away just when everything is ripe and ready to harvest here. On the stove, last week's mass of tomatoes simmers with herbs and garlic and a little wine. On the kitchen counter, today's tomatoes spread out and cover the white space with reds and a few yellowy oranges, ready to be eaten or canned or given away. This time, they'll go to neighbors because all I can fit into the few hours before I go is one batch of sauce.

And there are pears to think about. Out in the back field, they are dropping. Every day more litter the grass beneath the tree, and the deer and coyote and birds eat only some of them. Where animals have eaten, dripping bits of pear flesh are held on fallen leaves, and the bees and wasps buzz around the juicy remains. Every morning, I pick through the fallen ones, the tawny, rosy-skinned pears, and poke my hand through the damp grass to pull up the best. I carry them home in pockets that bulge. Now the pears wait in the kitchen, too. Will they last a week or more? Will I have time to make syrup this year? The seckle pears haven't started dropping yet. Maybe they'll wait until I'm home. But it's so hard to leave these here. I decide to take some with me to eat on the plane.

Everything is ripening so fast these days I am hard pressed to keep up. Vegetables in the garden and the wild fruits in the fields are clamoring to be gathered. And every day I find still more herbs to harvest. Yesterday I gathered hops near the ocean, and the low vines hang looped now over the rack in the herb room. This morning I plucked the strobiles by hand from some of the vines. The smell was wonderful—deep and cooling and mysterious somehow. I check the flowery fruits that are soaking in alcohol to make tincture. The liquid that is only hours old is dark brownish green, and will probably get lots darker. If the rest of the hops are dry when I get back, I'm going to make a wreath of them to hang over my bed. I've read that hops can be used in dream pillows to help with sleep. Maybe they'll work as well hanging up so I can smell them every night.

Kitchen Notes

I pluck more hops from the vines now, and spread them out in one layer on a cookie sheet. In the oven, they dry slowly and thoroughly, with the oven's heat driving out the last of moisture so they'll store well. The house smells terrific, and I feel myself relaxing just from the scent. Maybe I'll have a hops bath today—to soothe my frazzled and over-worked body before I leave.

Experiences with Hops

Mostly I use hops along with other herbs to help people with anxiety or nervousness. I use it especially with those who get stomach upsets when feeling tense, and it seems to smooth out rough edges in their lives—something we all can use once in a while!

FALL

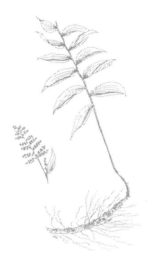

GENTIAN
Gentiana species

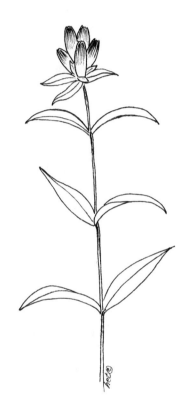

Reflections: Near the lake where I stand harvesting gentian, the flowers smile at me and we say hello to each other, and thank you. It is not so much that I say thank you out loud, or that they say thank you. We are just a thank you together. That's the way it always is—everything real is a thank you.

Description: The *Gentiana* species comprise a large group of wild-flowers found growing in damp woods and meadows. All species may be used interchangeably. In most species found in the North-east, the flowers are lavender to purple, and they have five petals. In most regional species, the leaves are opposite each other along the stem and form a whorl at the top of the plant just beneath the terminal flower cluster. Plant heights are up to 1¹/₂ feet.

The closed or bottle gentian, *Gentiana clausa,* has oval-shaped leaves, up to 4 inches long, with smooth margins and pointed tips. The deep blue tubular flowers are closed at the tip and look like long buds. The blossoms are up to 1¹/₂ inches long and occur at the top of the plant just beneath the terminal flower cluster. Plant heights are up to 1½ feet.

The fringe-tipped closed gentian, *G. andrewsii,* is very similar, but is fairly scarce. The blossoms of this species have fringes between the flower lobes that can be seen at the tip of the flower. The narrow-leaved gentian, *Gentiana linearis,* has similar flower parts, but with tips bent inward. The leaves are narrow and lance shaped. This species grows mainly in the North, in woods and meadows.

Stiff gentian, *G. quinquefolia,* has blossoms that are funnel shaped, with fringed tips. The flowers appear more open than the bottle species and are pinkish to lavender and occasionally white. The leaves are opposite, and upper leaves clasp the squarish stem.

Medicinal Uses: The primary medicinal use of the gentians is as an herbal bitter. The plant, taken before meals, will stimulate the flow of digestive juices, readying the body to digest and assimilate food eaten. Gentian stimulates the flow of saliva, bile, and gastric juices and thus aids in emptying the stomach. Gentian is especially useful with a heavy evening meal to aid in the digestive process when there is no chance for exercises afterward, or to relieve heartburn in cases where the digestive processes are weak.

Gentian has been used traditionally for poor appetite and chronic indigestion and flatulence. It is also good for short-term use in anorexia, following illness, or in the aged. Several of the compounds found in the gentians are anti-inflammatory, and therefore, it can also be used in mild fevers or in joint inflammations.

Harvesting: The whole plant is used. Pull up the plant, root and all, when it is in full flower. Since the fresh plant is strongest, a fresh-plant tincture is best for preserving its medicinal properties. To make the tincture, rinse soil from roots, chop all plant parts into ½ inch pieces, and place in alcohol for 2 weeks. To dry the plant for later use as a tea, rinse off soil, bundle stems together, and hang upside down in an airy place away from sun.

HARVESTING CAUTION: In some areas, some of the *Gentiana* species are at risk. Make certain to find out the status of the plant in your area before harvesting.

Dosages: Use 5–10 drops of the fresh-plant tincture in warm water 15–20 minutes before each meal. This mixture should be swished around the mouth as would a mouthwash, so that the bitter taste may activate the salivary glands. For tea, add $^1/_2$–1 tablespoon of fresh or dried chopped plant material to 1 cup of boiling water. Let steep 20 minutes.

CAUTION: Gentian used in excess may cause nausea, vomiting, and diarrhea. Dosages suggested should not be overdone.

FROM THE AUTHOR'S JOURNAL
SEPTEMBER 24

It's a perfect day. The sun is shining, the sky is blue, and only a few puffy white clouds edge the sky. A little breeze rustles the leaves of the sumacs, and the flowers sway in the garden. Everything is a riot of color and ripeness. All morning I work with herbs, cut and put away the dried things that have waited until I had time. Hops and raspberry leaves, horsetail and self-heal, blackberry leaves, and plantain all get tucked away for the season.

I stop after a while and drive over to the lake to see how the gentian is doing. It grows near the water, in a stand that edges the woods along the tiny dirt road. My timing is perfect. The gentians are all in full bud, some even beginning to fade a bit. The first time I saw it, I thought the plants were getting ready to bloom. But the field guides say that what appear to be buds are actually the full flower.

Today the newest blossoms are pale deep blue. As they get older, the flowers turn dark purple, and then start to collapse in on themselves a bit, browning at the edges. The blossoms stand in a cluster upon a whorl of leaves at the top of each plant, and each single stem has opposing leaves along its length. I chew on a leaf to check the flavor gentian is known for. The effect is not immediate, but as I chew the bitterness gets stronger, until I finally spit out the chewed bit.

Last year when I gathered gentian here I made a tincture. This time I'll be drying some for tea. I imagine it will be hard to drink, but I want to try more teas instead of using alcohol in everything. So, I'll experiment. I gather as many of the pretty plants as I can, and leave some to seed for future generations.

Down at the lake, a loon calls, loud and fast. She must feel threatened. I walk to the water to see what's happening, hoping to at least see the bird. Her call sounds like a mad, hysterical chuckle instead of the usual haunting cry. At the lake's edge, a small boat drifts through the bird's territory, and she quiets. She disappears then pops up again several feet away. It is too late in the season for her to be worried about a nest. I guess loons are just very private birds and don't like visitors.

The water is smooth and wide and dark blue with the sky's reflection. I rinse my fingers in it, and watch pebbles shift on the bottom with the slight motion.

On the way back to the car, I pick more gentian. Drooping overhead are ripe, purply-black, shiny elderberries, and I can't resist them. They can go for jelly, or for basket dye. I grab a bag from the car, snip the stems above the clusters, and pop them into the car next to the gentian. My fingers are stained as I drive home with the purple and blue treasures.

Experiences with Gentian

Recently I offered gentian to a young man who felt he was eating the right kinds of food, but was not getting the proper nutrients from what he ate. Gentian tea a few minutes before each meal seemed to help, and after a while he didn't seem to need it anymore.

Solomon's Seal
Smilacena racemosa and
Polygonatum biflorum

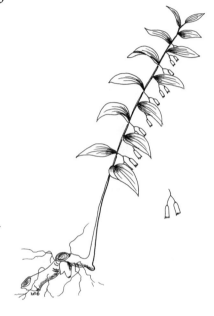

Reflections: Today I am out to harvest Solomon's seal. At 5:30 AM, the sky is still dark. Mars stands bright over the mountain ridge behind the house, and the fading moon casts enough light for me to walk into the woods to start my search. By the time light comes into the sky, I'm up to my elbows in dirt, pulling roots. When I lift a hand to take leaves out of my tangled hair, my fingers smell like earth.

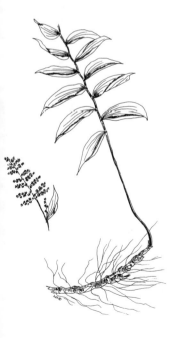

Description: The Solomon's seals are members of the Lily family, and while there are numerous varieties, two of them are used medicinally. Smooth Solomon's seal, *Polygonatum biflorum,* top, and false Solomon's seal, *Smilacena racemosa,* bottom, are used interchangeably. Both plants favor woodlands and grow in dry or damp woods or at the edges of forest along roadsides. They are sometimes planted in perennial or woodland gardens for ornamental purposes.

The roots of both plants are similar, being marked with round scars or "seals" where a leaf stalk has broken away from the root. In the smooth Solomon's seal, roots tend to be a bit darker, a golden cream color, and they exhibit heavier, knobbier seals than in the false Solomon's seal.

Both plants have leaves along a single, arched stem. Leaves of both plants are lance shaped and broad, and are up to 6 inches in length. Leaves are alternate in both species and have distinct parallel veins. The Solomon's seals may achieve 3 feet in height.

In the smooth Solomon's seal, the leaves are smooth on the surface and underneath. The blossoms appear from each leaf axil, dangling underneath the leaf pair. Blossoms are small, up to $^2/_3$ inch in length. And they are bell shaped with six flaring lobes at the tip. The flowers are pale greenish white in color and occur in clusters of two. The plant blooms in late spring and early summer.

The fruit develops from the dangling flowers and occurs as a dark bluish black berry hanging from the same leaf axils, generally in pairs. The berries are suspended from a thin green stalk, and occasionally the plant can be found with the stalks, even after the berries have dropped off.

In the false Solomon's seal, leaves are somewhat hairy along the margins and on the undersurfaces. The blossoms occur in a branched cluster at the terminal end of the stem. The cluster is roughly triangular in shape. Flowers are tiny, $^1/_8$ inch long, with three petals, and are ivory or white in color.

Fruit appears first as a translucent green berry mottled with pale, brownish red speckles. As the berries mature, they become bright translucent red. The fruit occurs in clusters at the terminal end of the stem, and the cluster forms a pyramidical or triangular shape as did the flowers earlier.

Medicinal Uses: The Solomon's seals are used interchangeably. The plants are demulcent and expectorant. They help soften mucus in the respiratory system, an important step in preventing congestion from causing an infection. In their function as expectorants, the Solomon's seals also help move mucus upward, facilitating its movement out of the body. These two actions can do much to keep symptoms of mild respiratory congestion from becoming a serious complication of a cold or influenza.

Harvesting: Dig roots of the Solomon's seals in the fall, after frosts have killed the foliage and leaves are brown and withered. Unearth the root, and wash carefully. Slice it into thin pieces, and spread to dry. Store when all moisture has been removed.

Dosages: A tablespoon of dried root simmered in $1\frac{1}{2}$ cups of boiling water for 15–30 minutes makes a decoction that can be drunk three times daily for relief of symptoms. Or the dried root can be simmered in equal its volume of honey to produce a syrup. Heat must be kept very low so the medicinal properties are not destroyed. This syrup can be taken three to four times daily, in doses of $\frac{1}{2}$–1 teaspoon.

FROM THE AUTHOR'S JOURNAL
SEPTEMBER 29

The air this morning is cold enough for several layers of clothing and for wool mittens to keep my hands warm. Down the road, everything stands in shadow. Just a sliver of light coming up lines the horizon in the east. From the back woods behind the house, an owl calls. One of my favorite things about walking these days is that I am out early enough in the dark to hear the owls. I stand for a while in the road, ear cocked to the woods, and listen, trying to place where the bird could be and wondering what little animal she stalks.

Down past Weeks's farm, it is too dark to see if the cows are out, but the farmer's bedroom light is on, so he must be getting ready to milk. In the woods next to the development road, I hear a rustling sound that gets louder and louder—something moving in the trees. I walk by and peer into the shadows, trying to see what's there, but scare myself with imaginings and move on. The rustling sounds approach the road. And when I look behind me, the telltale bright white stripes of a skunk glow in the moonlight and are moving quickly toward me. I walk faster still, talking all the while, explaining to the skunk that I am not a threat. By the time I am out of breath and up the hill, the skunk has turned off the road and disappeared.

The air smells cool and woodsy. Down the hill, all the new fall colors in the trees are lit up in the moonlight. It's a funny effect, like looking through a blue-black-green screen. Everything shimmers and glows.

Down Porter Road, lots of false Solomon's seal grows. Its leaves are papery now, and whatever berries the plants held are gone. Only the little stems underneath each leaf axil tell where the fruit used to be. I find a likely spot and start to dig. The leaf litter is thick and covers bouldery rocks that edge the stone wall. And when I jump on the shovel to give it a thrust home, it goes nowhere, and I fall off and my leg quivers for a while. There is barely any light to the morning yet, and finally I kneel to feel my way around to a good spot. When I can poke my fingers into the soil near a stem several inches all the way around, I decide to try digging again. This time the shovel goes in smoothly, and I dig deep to catch as much root as possible. Still, I miss some. These plants that grow near the stone wall have burrowed beneath and around rocks in the soil, and some plants seem to sprout from the very stones themselves. I walk into the woods and try there, and that goes easier.

Soon I have enough of this species, and start working on the smooth Solomon's seal, which grows right alongside its cousin in this open place. The berries on these plants are a clear translucent red color and stand at the end of the curving stems. The plants have bigger roots, too, and the roots go deeper and soon I am covered with dirt and leaf litter.

Kneeling on the side of the road in the pale morning, half-buried in soil, suddenly I am caught by the headlights of the school bus that comes rumbling by. I scurry into a sitting position and pat my hair into place, hoping to look normal. For a while afterward, I imagine being arrested for loitering on a deserted roadside in the dark, but no one comes to get me, so I keep working.

When the bag is full, sun has just begun to peek over the horizon. I pat the soil back into place and stamp around on it. Finally, I pluck dead leaves from my sweater before walking home.

Kitchen Notes

At home I clean the roots under running water. Each root has lots of round, bumpy places, the "seals," along its length. Roots of the two species are similar, but the false roots are bone white, while the smooth roots are creamy, almost golden white. When the soil is washed away, I slice the roots thinly. Some of the roots have thin, kinky rootlets sprouting from them, and the slices look like white spidery insects. I spread them out on a screen for drying.

Experiences with Solomon's Seal

Every year Solomon's seal roots go into honey for a cough syrup. The taste is woodsy-spicy, and even the kids think it makes a delicious medicine. We use it to relieve congestion and minor coughs, and count on it every winter to get us through the season of colds and flu.

Yellow Dock
Rumex crispus

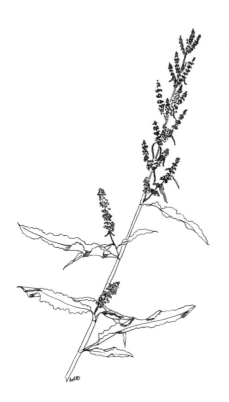

Reflections: This morning the air smells damp and cold and is full of the scents of the tanned and dying leaves that line the road. Crows call across the field and in the maple tree grackles chatter and squawk. Chickadees at the feeder make their little noises and then dive down to eat. The morning is gray—a good fall day, good for tucking in and good for transitions. Out in the field, yellow dock has new green leaves at its base, sprouting even as the winter comes on. I think what a joy this plant is— so common that we barely notice it, yet providing us with so much.

Description: Considered a common weed, yellow dock is also known as curly dock, a name that refers to its wavy-margined leaves. Yellow dock is not particular about soils and can be found commonly along roadsides and in fields and waste places.

The root is pale to dark yellow inside, with a reddish brown outer bark. The leaves of yellow dock are alternate and very long at the base of the plant, up to 1 foot, getting progressively smaller near the top. They are lance shaped with pointed tips and have very wavy leaf margins. Plant height is up to 6 feet.

The flowers of this Buckwheat family member are small and greenish, up to about $1/6$ inch in length. They grow in long, branched clusters atop the central stem, and flower parts generally inconspicuous unless examined very closely. The plant blooms June through September.

Fruit forms from the blossoms and occurs along the same branched terminal clusters. The brownish red fruit is formed of three distinct sides, as is typical of Buckwheat family members. Clusters of fruit, which can be seen on the plant well into winter and the following spring, are one of the distinguishing features of the plant.

Medicinal Uses: The root of yellow dock has a number of uses. It is known traditionally as a blood purifier and has been used for its ability to help the body break down and eliminate toxins. Yellow dock works on the liver, promoting the flow of bile and other digestive juices and it is one of the herbs that can be used in helping to balance the liver functions after a bout of hepatitis. It can be used alone, as a tea or tincture, or with other herbs.

Because of its action as a cholagogue, yellow dock can be used as a remedy for gallbladder complaints, where it helps stimulate the flow of bile and aid in relieving congestion.

Yellow dock is also somewhat laxative, although gentle in action. It can be used for chronic constipation, where it will work gently but effectively. Yellow dock can be used where there is poor digestion of fats or metabolism of proteins. It is especially helpful in skin disturbances such as psoriasis, eczema, or acne, where it helps cleanse the body and eliminate waste products. Externally, yellow dock can be used as a skin application for infections, ulcers, or cysts.

Harvesting: The root of yellow dock should be dug in the fall when the fruit is dry and reddish brown in color. The roots will be distinctly yellow. Wash roots carefully, and slice healthy roots into thin pieces. Spread out to dry on appropriate material, and store when thoroughly dried.

Dosages: Yellow dock is fairly water soluble, and the herb may be taken as a tea or in tincture form. To use the tea, make a decoction by placing 1 tablespoon of the root into 1 cup of water, and bring to a boil. Simmer on low heat for 10–15 minutes, and then strain out plant material. Drink the tea three times a day. A tincture, made with fresh or dried plant material, can be taken in 30 drop doses three times daily.

FROM THE AUTHOR'S JOURNAL
OCTOBER 10

This morning I walk along the road carrying a shovel and bags to harvest yellow dock. Down by the house where the porcupines live, it grows in abundance, and now its three-sided flowers are dark and brownish red—gone to seed. I sniff at the air as I walk. The earth scents are starting to disappear. That's what I miss most in winter—the earthy smells. Now there is dew and cold, and a dark, deep scent from the damp bark of trees, and at the farm, the sweet scent of cows and hay and chimney smoke. But the green and flowery smells are going.

By the time I get to the house where yellow dock stands, there is just enough light to see green. Low evening primrose grows, and wide, fresh-looking plantain leaves, and some low clover. I walk in a bit before I find a healthy-looking dock plant and start digging.

The earth here is loose and dark and smells delightful. The roots I turn up are fat, long, and yellow when I scrape away the outer bark. I work on a few plants, one after another, choosing good spots. While I work, gunshots echo against the mountain. Surely it's not hunting season already? This is the time of day—early, with little light yet—when hunters set out for deer. I didn't think it was time yet, though, and I worry for the animals.

My bag fills with yellow dock. I stop and look at the roots. They are long and thick. Some of the plants have roots that are black and weak and seem rotten, so I break these off. When I get home, I'll separate out the healthy ones from those that seem damaged and keep just the good ones. I think somehow that the darkest yellow ones are the most medicinal, but I'm not sure. Maybe I just like them because they seem so robust. I'd like to stay and work here all day, but the air is chilly. Birds chatter anxiously, and the western sky darkens, threatening rain. I race home with my bag of roots, trying to stay warm and dry.

Kitchen Notes

In the kitchen, I clean the roots and then begin to chop them up. The long, thin ones are easy. They are almost rubbery, and each slice reveals pale yellow insides. The thicker roots are woody and harder to cut. I tangle with them, and remember how much work roots are. But the work is worth it. The thick, hard-bodied roots are beautiful—dark, with concentric circles of yellow that gets almost orange near the center. These roots smell deep and dark and a little bitter, and a kind of stinging smell rises from the bowl I put them in.

I spread the bright slices out on screens to dry, clean up the kitchen, and get ready for work.

Experiences with Yellow Dock

I first learned of yellow dock from a friend who used a poultice of the root to help relieve a cyst. It worked within a day or so, she said. She managed to avoid surgery that way and the cyst has never recurred. Yellow dock is one of the herbs I use, too, in formulas for people with skin problems such as psoriasis or eczema, and it also helps for severe acne. I've also given yellow dock to several friends who suffer from constipation. They found it to work gently and reliably. So many uses form a plant we disdain as a weed. Surely there's a lesson in that!

Witch Hazel
Hamamelis virginiana

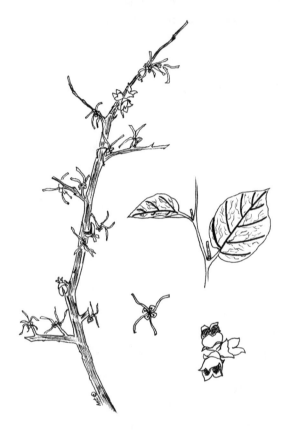

Reflections: The air is cool and full of scent. I lean down to pick a bright green wintergreen berry and stand up to bump my head on a tree limb. Untangling my hair from it, I catch a glimpse of yellow and step back to discover witch hazel all in flower. What a joy to find these plants blooming when all else is dying down for winter's rest. I pick a few of the twigs to take along with me and see an eensy spider dangling from one of them. I carefully put him back on a smooth-barked branch of his tree before I walk home.

Description: Witch hazel is a small tree or shrub. It favors damp woods and may be found along some roadsides that border forest areas. Witch hazel is somewhat unique in that its yellow blossoms appear in fall just as the leaves are being shed. And it can frequently be found with its bare branches decorated by spidery yellow blossoms.

The leaves of the shrub or tree are dark, dull green in color on the surface, and paler underneath. They are egg shaped or oval, with wavy, toothed margins and distinct, straight vein patterns. The younger leaves may be somewhat downy. A distinctive feature of the leaf is its uneven base, with one side being definitely shortened. Leaves are up to 5 inches long, and about half as wide and may be found along bare twigs in autumn and into winter.

Witch hazel fruit occurs as a hard, roundish capsule that contains shiny black seeds. The capsule splits when mature, and the sides fold back into four sharply curved points. Seeds are flung through the air with an audible popping sound. Empty seed capsules may be found on the branches into winter, along with the remains of blossoms.

Medicinal Uses: Witch hazel leaves, twigs, and bark are used for their astringent, anodyne, and hemostatic properties. These attributes make it useful for minor wounds, scratches, and insect bites. It helps reduce inflammation and tone injured tissues, thereby speeding the healing process. A wash of witch hazel can also help reduce or control a mild poison ivy reaction. It can offer some relief, too, for the pain and inflammation of sunburns. Witch hazel can be helpful for tired, irritated eyes. Used externally as a poultice over the closed lids, a wash of the herb can be counted on for reducing symptoms brought on by eyestrain.

Witch hazel has been used for centuries as an external application for cosmetic purposes. Its astringency makes it useful in toning the skin. If the tendency to form pimples or blackheads exists, it will help to cleanse and close pores and act as an antiseptic, helping to prevent infection of skin eruptions. A wash of witch hazel is also an old-time external application for varicose vein flare-ups. As a salve, it can also be counted on for aid in hemorrhoids, where its hemostatic action helps lessen bleeding and its astringency works to tighten tissues.

Internally, witch hazel can be used like other astringent herbs as a tea to help relieve mild diarrhea.

Harvesting: The leaves and small twigs of witch hazel are gathered throughout the growing season, spring through early fall. Pluck individual leaves from the tree, or cut small, leaf-bearing twigs. Spread individual leaves to dry on screens, paper bags, or baskets, and store when crumbly. Bundle twigs at the stem base, and hang upside down to dry. To use witch hazel bark, strip in small patches from the tree in early spring when the leaves are just sprouting. Avoid stripping bark from around the tree in a complete circle. Spread out pieces of bark, cut when fully dry, and store for later use.

Dosages: To use internally, make a tea of witch hazel using 1 tablespoon of dried leaves, twigs, or bark to 1 cup of boiling water. Steep 20–30 minutes, and drink three times daily for diarrhea.

For external use, make a strong tea of dried plant parts, and pat on injured area several times a day. Or pour the strong tea over a cloth, and apply directly to the injured or affected skin. Repeat this treatment several times daily. For irritated or tired eyes, use a compress soaked in strong witch hazel tea, apply to closed lids, and rest for 10–15 minutes. Repeat several times daily if necessary. For skin wounds and irritations or for insect bites or hemorrhoids, witch hazel can be added to salves and applied several times a day.

FROM THE AUTHOR'S JOURNAL
OCTOBER 15

Walking down the development road this Saturday morning, I am out to see the colors. Because this is a new road, and because so much was cleared out early in spring, there are lots of baby trees. Each and every tiny tree is scarlet and crimson and flame red. The field is ablaze with color. Far beyond, the lake is full of sunrise. I stand and turn and look in every direction, breathing deeply. What an incredible season fall is! I walk farther down the hill and glance toward the raspberry vines where the young fox hid in summer and then followed alongside me, checking me out. This morning there is nothing there.

On the other side of the road, where grass is sparse and smooth and not much grows, sweet fern has started to sprout. Single stems of it poke up into the air, full of dark leaves. At the bend in the road, near the bottom of the hill, coyote scat lies, and where soft sandy earth sinks away from the road there are tracks. I bend to see them closer and guess that they are coyote. I press my fingers into the deep impressions, trying to remember exactly how dog tracks differ. There is something about the outer toes, but I'm not sure what and will have to look it up when I get home.

I walk farther, keeping an eye on the growth that is turning colors. Ferns are brown and crumply. Raspberry leaves are reddish around some edges and on their way to purple. Some are still green—the low ones—and other low stuff is green, too. Sorrels and new bristly stemmed sarsaparilla have sprouted in the mild days, maybe thinking it was spring again.

At the little waterway, cattail leaves are yellowy, and the brown spikes are fluffy and overgrown. Some of the seeds in the packed spikes have started to blow away in the wind, making the spikes look scruffy. Lush growth around the water has faded back, and the stream looks wider, too, with the curves of the hills starting to show.

The air is cool and full of the scent of wintergreen, and as I lean down to pick a bright wintergreen berry, I am surprised to see witch hazel in bloom. I didn't realize it was time for it to flower yet. Most of the branches are bare of leaves, and the yellow flowers that look like scraggly starbursts poke out from bare gray bark all along the branches. There are a few coarse leaves, and they are yellowing, getting ready to fall. They feel thick and stiff, and on their undersides is a thin fuzz. The leaf veins are rather prominent, deep, and the leaf surfaces are glossy. The characteristic that marks witch hazel for me is the uneven leaf bases. One side of each leaf is distinctly shorter than the other. Along the branches where flowers stand, there are a few brown, oddly shaped capsules that hold small, dark seeds. I remember hearing that the seeds actually spring out of the capsules when disturbed by wind or animals, and they fly long distances from the tree. But I've never seen that happen.

The witch hazel flowers are pretty, and I pick a few twigs to take home with me. Now that I've found this place where witch hazel grows, I think how much fun it will be to make my very own supply of extract. Maybe in the spring I'll come back for the new growth of bark. For now, I bundle up the pretty twigs and take them home through the flaming woods.

Experiences with Witch Hazel

I've used a wash of witch hazel as a simple astringent for cuts and scratches. I offer it, too, to teenagers with acne. Cleansing the face with a little witch hazel wash on a cotton ball or gauze a couple of times a day helps keep the skin fresh and clean, especially on those hot and sticky summer days. I also use witch hazel along with other herbs in a douche formula for vaginal yeast infections. And lately I've suggested witch hazel packs for a woman with varicose veins, and she found it helpful.

Skunk Cabbage
Symplocarpus foetidus

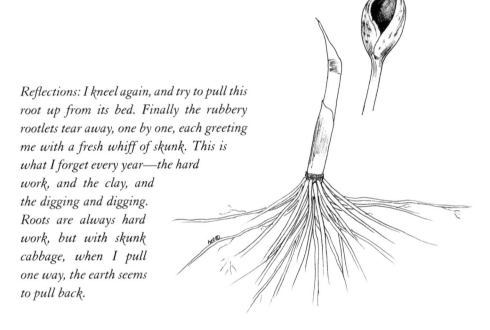

Reflections: I kneel again, and try to pull this root up from its bed. Finally the rubbery rootlets tear away, one by one, each greeting me with a fresh whiff of skunk. This is what I forget every year—the hard work, and the clay, and the digging and digging. Roots are always hard work, but with skunk cabbage, when I pull one way, the earth seems to pull back.

Description: Skunk cabbage is one of the first wildflowers to emerge in spring when the warmth of its growth actually melts the snow covering it. It grows in wet woodlands, swamps, and marshes and along damp streambeds. The roots grow very deep to anchor the plant in the mucky soil in which it grows, and the leaves, blossom, and root emit a strong skunklike odor when the plant is disturbed or damaged.

Skunk cabbage blossoms appear before leaves erupt and are often inconspicuous, half-buried in muck or pushing up through dead, wet leaves. The single flower is odd shaped and unusual. The exterior flower part is a hoodlike spathe shaped like two cupped hands or an almost enclosed seashell. The color is a mottling of reddish-or purplish brown on yellow-green. The interior flower part is a knobby spadix that is often seen covered with powdery yellow pollen. The bloom grows up to 6 inches in height, and it appears from late February through May.

The leaves first begin to appear as a tightly rolled spike that pushes up next to the flower and later unfurls to reveal several very large, roundish, dark green leaves. Later in the season, the leaves form a carpet over the ground. They may be up to 2 feet in length and almost as wide. They are heavily veined and arise directly from the ground with no apparent stalk. Plant height may be up to 1 foot, and leaves are visible through the first frost.

Medicinal Uses: A preparation of the root of skunk cabbage is expectorant, antispasmodic, stimulant, and diaphoretic. These properties make it useful in conditions such as asthma or bronchitis, where it will help relax the bronchial mucosa and promote a free flow of mucus. Skunk cabbage can also help reduce a fever by producing a sweat, and this factor makes it helpful in colds or flu where elevated temperature is a problem. Skunk cabbage can be used in any kind of spasmodic or nervous coughing and can be taken as a tea, tincture, or powder.

Harvesting: The root should be dug in the fall after the first frost has killed leaf material. It is best to identify the plant in early spring, because in the fall the leaves begin to die back and the plant can be hard to recognize. Mark each plant you have identified with brightly colored string or twine, and be certain of your identification. Find the skunk cabbage plants that bear distinctive, low growing flowers, and have a characteristic skunk scent, and mark only these plants. Then, in the fall, gather and use only those plants that you have marked and which smell strongly of skunk.

Once the skunk cabbage roots have been dug, clean them, slice into small, thin pieces, and spread out to dry. The fresh roots can also be used to make a fresh-plant tincture.

HARVESTING CAUTION: Another plant, green hellebore, begins to sprout in the same mucky places just as skunk cabbage is coming up, and it is highly toxic and fatal if ingested. The two plants are often both called skunk cabbage in New England states, making the distinction even more difficult.

Dosages: For tea, use $^1/_2$ teaspoon of dried root to 1 cup of boiling water, and let steep for 20 minutes. Drink three times daily. Skunk cabbage can also be taken in powder form. To use it this way, powder the dried root, weigh the powder, and mix it with ten times its weight in honey. Mix thoroughly, and take $^1/_2$ teaspoon of the mixture three times daily. For dried-plant tincture, use 5–10 drops of tincture three times daily.

CAUTION: Some people have allergic reactions to skunk cabbage, and it is best to take only a very small dose for the first few times. It should be avoided altogether by people who have sensitivities to many substances.

FROM THE AUTHOR'S JOURNAL
OCTOBER 15

I go down to the lake, to a swampy place where skunk cabbage and fiddleheads are the first green to come up after snow melts. From the road, I stop to look at the little pond that spills into the stream. In spring, the whole surface of the water is covered with the wide green leaves of skunk cabbage. Now, the water is dark and low and not much stirs. There are some spiky plant stems poking up from the water, but they are black and soft and I can't even see where skunk cabbage stood. I walk around through the woods to look for plants to harvest.

The forest floor is carpeted with fallen leaves Partridgeberry is full of red berries and grows over mossy tree roots that stick up from the soft earth. At the edge of the little pond, I look again for skunk cabbage and find nothing that looks familiar. I walk farther, treading the streambank, thinking that if I follow the water, surely I'll find skunk cabbage.

No one has walked here for a long time. Tiny invisible spiderwebs net little branches together, and they catch on my nose and in my hair and eyelashes. I brush at them with a hand and then wipe an arm across my face to get rid of them. Finally I walk with the shovel in front of me and it clears a path so I stop getting webby.

At the narrow stream's edge, I stop again to check. Golden leaves float on the dark surface of the water and moss holds the earth in place. At my feet, one wide blackened leaf is translucent, crumply, and almost unrecognizable. But at its base, just protruding from the earth, is a knobby curve of what looks like a skunk cabbage flower. I put in the shovel, step hard on it, and a clod of clay separates from the stream-bank. The smell that drifts up gives me my answer—skunk! I work some more, until the rubbery white rootlets are exposed, and then reach through the muck with my fingers and pull. The rootlets are long and fat, and there is a thicker main root that breaks off into my hand. I pat the clod of clay back into place, rearrange the moss cover, and move on to find more.

Now that I've seen skunk cabbage once, it is easier to spot. At another curve of the streambank, I try again, hoping to get a whole root. This place is higher, not so wet, but the soil is still solid clay. When the shovel tilts to lift up the roots, the earth pulls back with loud sucking noises. After a few rounds, I pull up the soil with my hands and see a ring of white snaky rootlets. They grow outward from the underground stem in a pretty circle. I trace underneath them, feeling for the main root, and find it deep beneath the clay. I have to admire this plant, clinging so tightly to its home. Maybe its tenacious hold keeps the slippery muck from being washed away by the water that moves through.

Finally, I have enough of this root, and enough of the hard work. If I need more, there is lots of it here, and I can come back. Now, I have gluey, black earth all over my hands and up to my elbows. My knees are wet and black, and my shirtsleeves are dark with muck. I grab the shovel and bag of smelly roots, and walk back to the car, hoping no one will see—or smell—me. I almost forget to stop and thank the earth for its gift, and thank the skunk cabbage, too. I stand still for a while, and smile, and then walk through the woods to my car.

Experiences with Skunk Cabbage

I haven't used skunk cabbage much. The first time I gathered it, I put a fresh piece of root on my tongue, and the prickly, burning sensation was intense and lasted for quite a while. Since then, I've met a woman who takes the herb every year in powder form and says it works fine for her. Maybe this year I'll give it a try. Maybe if I dry the root, it won't taste quite so acrid.

BAYBERRY
Myrica pensylvanica and species

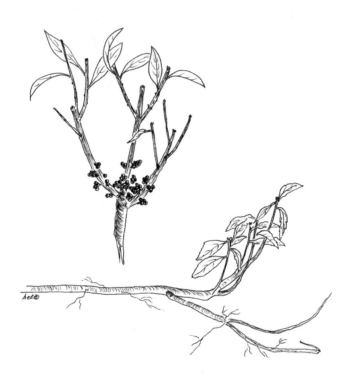

Reflections: On the floor next to the kitchen table are several bags of herbs harvested on the little island. Lily of the valley roots wait to be processed, along with a bag of fat rose hips. Another sack is filled with bayberry full of waxy blue seed. The scent of the crushed leaves is wonderful, and the roots are cool, sandy, and sharp smelling. So much wonderful work to do!

Description: Bayberry is a shrub or small tree found in sandy soil, often along seacoasts or in sandy swamps where it thrives on moist conditions. The leaves, bark, and fruit are highly aromatic when crushed.

The leaves are up to 3 inches long and 1 inch wide and are somewhat leathery and thickened. They are lance shaped, with some toothing, and they occur alternately along the gray branches. Leaves are shiny green on the surface and paler underneath. When crushed, they emit a strong, aromatic scent. Plant height is up to 6 feet.

Bayberry flowers are tiny and occur in small clusters at the base of the leaf. They are greenish yellow in color and can be found in early spring.

The fruit is a small, roundish berry with a bumpy surface that is caused by the coating of bluish white wax. Fruit can be found on the plant late summer to fall and through the winter. It is aromatic when crushed.

Medicinal Uses: The root bark of bayberry is the primary medicinal part of the plant. Bark from the stems may also be used, as well as the berries. Bayberry is highly astringent and works on the mucous membranes, especially those of the stomach, intestinal tract, and sinuses. It also acts as a stimulant, increasing blood flow to the mucous membranes. These qualities make it useful in such conditions as sore throat or bleeding gums, where bayberry works to tone tissues and reduce swelling. It is also helpful in chronic sinus infections or inflammations where it will reduce swelling of the membranes and help cut down on discharge. Taken at the first signs of a cold, bayberry can act as a diaphoretic and help reduce fever as well as relieve symptoms.

Because of its action in the intestinal tract, bayberry can be used in cases of stomach or intestinal ulceration. It increases circulation to the area while acting to tone tissues involved. Bayberry is a specific remedy for colitis.

Harvesting: Dig the plant up in fall after the first frosts. Remove roots from the branches, and rinse off soil. Strip bark from the root. It is helpful to pound the roots first to loosen the bark and make it easier to peel away. Dry the bark by spreading it out on appropriate material, and keep in a well-ventilated place for 1 to 2 weeks. When all bark is brittle, store.

Dosages: To use bayberry as a tea, make a decoction by placing 1 tablespoon of root bark in a pan with 1 cup of water. Bring to a boil, simmer on low heat for 15–20 minutes, and then strain out plant parts. Drink the tea three times daily. A tincture may be used in doses of 30–60 drops, taken three times daily. If using the dried berries, chew four or five dried fruit three times a day.

FROM THE AUTHOR'S JOURNAL
OCTOBER 17

I am out on a tiny island to get bayberry. There hasn't been much rain since last time I was here, and all the growth is stunted. Soil that is already sandy is "dry as a bone" and blows around in any breeze. When a car moves by, a cloud of dust marks its passage for a long, long time.

A friend and I walk the island, picking rose hips that are soft and plumply ripe. We find bayberry, too, growing in huge hedges all along the shore. Last year's growth holds waxy berries, pale blue and fragrant when we crush them. I decide to collect some for candle making, and fill a pocket. The leaves are stiff and smooth edged, and smell delightful, and I break off twigs full of leaves and berries to take home. A hard wind whips the ocean over nearby rocks and the spray sprinkles us while we work. All the scents—the spicy bayberry leaves, sweet and fruity rose hips, the salt air, and the dryness of sandy soil—are almost dizzying.

We leave the shore and go inland a bit. Along every road or path bayberry grows, starting small then rising into bushes. We decide to begin with the little plants that edge a narrow dirt road. I use a shovel at first, but it is hardly needed. The bayberry pulls up easily and I trace through the dry, sandy soil with my fingers to follow the root path. One tiny plant leads to another larger one and then to a clump of bushes, on and on. We could pull up much of the roadside if we tried. It makes me think how important these plants are, holding down the island's loose and sandy soil.

As we cut the roots, a sharp and distinct smell drifts up, nothing much like the bayberry fragrance of the leaves or bruised berries. I taste a bit of root, and it is instantly astringent, so sharp it's hard to keep chewing. The flavor is a little bitter, but the most intense sensation is the astringency, puckering my tongue and lips.

The roots are easy to gather, and the bag fills fast, but we barely make a dent in the roadside population. The sandy soil falls easily back into place. We pat it down, dust ourselves off, and gather bayberry and rose hips to take home.

Kitchen Notes

The bayberry roots have to be processed right away. What I need from them is the root bark, and if they sit too long, the roots will stiffen and be hard to cut. I separate twigs from roots and grab a knife and bowl and cutting board and get set to work. The roots are mostly long and narrow. One is thick, knobby, and irregular. The soil on them rinses off easily under water.

Getting the bark from the roots is hard work. I pound at one root with a big knife handle and the bark flakes away. It is easier to cut now, but there are lots of roots with lots of bark to strip. After an hour or so, the bark chips add up. I pick them up in cupped hands, and sniff at them, and the same sharp astringent scent is evident. I put the flakes into a jar and press them down to compact them. Grain alcohol goes over them, and a little stone; they will sit for a couple of weeks, making tincture.

The table is a litter of root bits that can go to the compost. Some of the stems bear pale blue, waxy berries. I pull them off to save, and gather the leftover roots and stems to take outside. The air inside the kitchen smells delightful, sweet from the rose hips drying, and sharp and pungent from the bayberry. What lovely scents to flavor the day!

DANDELION
Taraxacum officinale

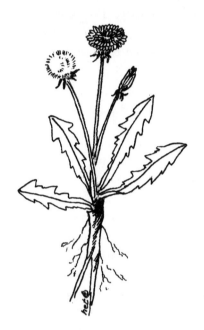

Reflections: In the kitchen I work on bits of dandelion root. It's strange that we curse this plant's intrusion in our lawns, and meanwhile it goes on undeterred, offering food and first color in the spring and simple medicine for so many ills. It helps remind me that the truest things are simple—there for us whether we notice them or not. Out in the back field, the coyotes bay and chant together. The sounds move back toward the forest, leaving everything quiet. And the moon shines on.

Description: Dandelion is a common weed of lawns, fields, and roadsides. The plants are abundant throughout much of the United States. When torn or crushed, the leaves and flower stalks release a white, milky juice.

The leaves arise from the base of the plant and are up to 16 inches long. They are deeply lobed, and the margins are irregularly toothed. Leaves may be found green and healthy-looking from earliest spring through late fall and into winter. Dandelion may grow up to 1¹/₂ feet in height.

The flower heads are bright yellow and are composed of numerous ray petals. The blossoms are up to 2 inches wide, and each forms atop a central stem that arises from the base of the plant. Bracts at the base of the flower head are turned downward. Dandelion can be found in bloom early spring through late fall. Dandelion fruit occurs as a seed attached to long, silky hairs that develop to form the familiar white seed head found on the plant as it matures.

Medicinal Uses: The root of dandelion has properties that make it useful for variety of complaints. Dandelion is diuretic and provides potassium at the same time. It is thus an ideal remedy for the fluid retention of heart problems or PMS, since it will help maintain proper chemical balance while allowing elimination of excess water and waste products from the body. Dandelion can also be used preventively in the tendency to form kidney stones or gravel.

Dandelion root is known as a liver tonic and cholagogue, and it has been used traditionally for liver congestion or digestive sluggishness or in the jaundice that lingers after hepatitis. Dandelion may be used supportively in diabetes, because of its action on the liver. It is one of the herbs that can be used, too, in therapies for chronic skin problems, such as psoriasis or eczema. Dandelion also has a history of use in gallstones or chronic gallbladder inflammations since the root stimulates the flow of bile. In addition, dandelion root is mildly laxative, and it can be helpful in chronic constipation, especially of the aged, where it works gently but dependably. Dandelion has no known toxicity and can be safely depended on in tea or tincture form.

Harvesting: Dig the root either very early in the spring, just as leaf sprouts are showing, or in the fall after several frosts have killed back leafy material. Clean well, and slice into thin pieces. Spread these out to dry on screens, baskets, or paper bags, and when all pieces are dry, store for later use.

Dosages: To make tea, place 1–2 tablespoons of dried root into 1$\frac{1}{2}$ cups of boiling water. Simmer gently on low heat for 20–30 minutes, and then strain out plant material. Drink 1 cup of the decoction three times daily. If using the tincture, $^1/_2$–1 teaspoon of tincture may be taken three times a day.

I am out on a chilling October afternoon to plant bulbs. It has been a month or so since the garden faded, and just enough time has passed to make me eager to work in the earth once more before winter closes in. For a long time, all I am is the digging and shifting of clumps of sod, and the sifting of soil through fingers. Fifty or a hundred bulbs get tucked into cold soil, and my hands grow numb with burrowing. Finally, all the bulbs are in. When I gather myself to go, I have worked through the dusk and into the night. The full moon bobs just above the horizon, lighting the yard.

I stand and just watch for a while, unable to go inside. Instead, I decide to gather the dandelion roots that stand in the field behind the garden. I trudge back through the yard that is lit with moonlight, and find the dandelions gone to seed. Their heads poke up around the field's edge. Here, where calendula still bends, dry and brittle, and where tomatoes and melons and broccoli flourished, now there is dandelion to do.

I start digging, and unearth huge clumps of roots tangled together. Holding the clumps in my lap, I separate one root from another, tracing a finger along each path of rootlets to its source and shaking it free. The roots smell dense and sharp. To make sure everything I gather is dandelion, I snap off pieces of root and watch the milky juice squeeze out. The pieces taste bitter, and gritty.

I dig forever in the cold night, hauling up as many roots as I can before my hands grow numb. Still, I am reluctant to go in. The moon lights up the field, the faded garden, the fruit trees, the house, and throws blue shadows. Finally, I bundle up the roots to take inside. Just as I open the door, coyotes appear in the field. They come every evening for the dropped apples and pears. Tonight I feel a kinship with them—we harvest the earth's offerings together. When I am in, they begin to sing.

Kitchen Notes

Inside the kitchen, I clutter the counter with dirty roots, scattering clods of soil and sticky latex. The roots get cleaned under running water. Old leaves are broken from each plant, and then the roots get scrubbed with a vegetable brush, and rinsed again. I gather tools—a sharp knife, a pan for the clean roots, a large jar with its lid; then the alcohol goes over them; and finally a clean, smooth stone to keep them down. Once the tincture is assembled, it goes into the herb cabinet to sit for a while. The rest of the root I spread out on baskets where it will dry for tea.

Experiences with Dandelion

Last year's supply of dandelion went for several purposes. I offered it to a woman at work for help with a blood pressure problem. She wanted something simple to take and knew dandelion would act as a diuretic. Since then, she uses dandelion routinely. Now she no longer needs to use potassium supplements, and finds that her blood pressure has remained stable, and lower than it was. I also gave some to a neighbor who used is for the bloating she got with PMS. She used it in the few days before her period started, and found it helpful. Another friend's sister took dandelion root in a formula along with other herbs to help her recover from hepatitis. Lately I've been wanting to try it for help with blood sugar control in diabetics. Since dandelion works on the liver and is safe to take, it seems like a good bet in those cases. So many uses for such a commonplace plant!

Rose Hips
Rosa species

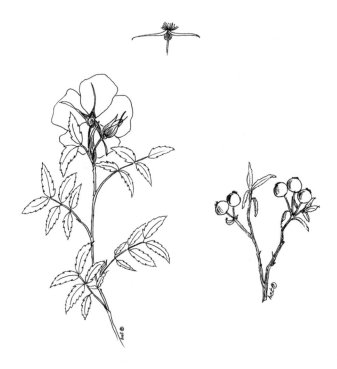

Reflections: In this early morning, the room's light throws bright reflections against the wide window that closes out the dark. I can see myself, and the flashy, flowery wallpaper, and the fern, and all the bits and scraps of rose hips in a clutter. Out the very top of the window, in just one space of dark the kitchen light can't reach, a bright star twinkles in the sky. The room is fragrant with rose hips drying in the oven, and I get ready to make a tea of the rosy fruit.

Description: Roses are familiar thorny-stemmed, ornamental shrubs, usually with fragrant blooms. A number of rose species have escaped from early gardens and grow in the wild. While various species prefer different growing locations and soil types, wild roses are common to roadsides and fields and along the seashore. All may be used for the same medicinal purposes.

Rose leaves are divided into five to eleven leaflets that occur along a spiny stem. In some species, leaves appear wrinkly. The leaf margins are toothed, and leaves are between 1 and 6 inches long. The plant grows from 1 to 8 feet in height.

The flowers are quite pretty, with five regular petals that are $^1/_4$ inch wide. Colors range from white to lavender pink. The plant blooms in summer and into fall. Fruit is a red, fleshy hip that contains many seeds. It is edible when ripe.

Medicinal Uses: Rose petals are astringent, and like most herbs with the same property, can be relied upon to provide some aid in mild diarrhea. The petals have also been used in skin preparations, where their soothing astringency helps to reduce inflammation of tissue and provide some tone. Rose petal tea can also be used as a pleasant gargle and mouthwash for sore throats. A wash made of rose petals has also been traditionally used as a treatment for irritated or tired eyes.

The fruit, known as rose hips, contains a high amount of vitamin C. Although some of the vitamin content is lost in drying and processing, rose hip tea does provide some nutrition and is a healing aid in colds and influenza.

Harvesting: Gather petals when the flower is in full bloom and spread to dry on screens or cheesecloth in a location where ventilation is optimal and light is low. To harvest rose hips, wait until the first of fall frosts have turned the hips bright crimson. Gather, and process immediately. The larger hips should be halved and the seeds and small hairs removed. If humidity is very low, and days are warmish, the smaller fruit may dry adequately by being spread on screens. Otherwise, spread one layer thick on cookie sheets, and place on the middle rack of an oven. Set temperature to its lowest setting, and prop the oven door open to allow moisture to escape. Dry for several hours, and when thoroughly dried, cool and store.

Dosages: To use rose hips, make an infusion with 1–2 tablespoons of hips to 1 cup of boiling water. Let steep 10–20 minutes, strain, and drink several times a day. Rose petals can be used as a tea or wash, using 1–2 teaspoons of dried petals to 1 cup of boiling water, and should be steeped for 10 minutes.

FROM THE AUTHOR'S JOURNAL
OCTOBER 29

I drive to the ocean to get away and do something different, and to gather rose hips. Near the water, huge green hedges are speckled with bright fruit. The hedges form a wall against the beach, and then spread into a thick blanket that covers the sandy earth and runs right up to any structure. The fruits are bright and scarlet, and the past few days of cold have ripened them.

I poke a hand into the mass of wrinkly leaves and reach for a rose hip, but a wind jiggles everything and I get stuck a few times first. Once the wind slows, the work is better. The hips come off the bushes easily. They are just barely soft to the touch, and their scent makes my mouth water.

I chew a bit of the bright fruit away from its seeds and it tastes delicious—sweet and tangy. Some hips taste like a combination of plum and ripe persimmon, while others are more like very ripe tomatoes. At first the seeds get in the way, but I keep practicing and get better. I nibble around the sides to get the ripest flesh, then nibble at the base and suck the whole hip without biting into the ivory mass of seeds.

There are so many hips I lose track of time and am just this process of stealing one hip and then another from its thorns. Then the sky turns dark and fierce, and the wind gets forceful, blowing and blowing, and my hands get stiff with cold. I stand on the beach, on the million gray rocks smooth and round from the beating waves, with dried seaweed at my feet. Then the wind blows so hard it tips me over and I laugh and smile and close my eyes and sniff long breaths of ocean, salt, and seaweed.

When the rain finally starts, I unfold my frozen limbs and carry the bag of bright fruit back to the car.

Kitchen Notes

At the kitchen table, I work on the fat rose hips. I split them in half, and scoop out the hard seeds. The hips are plump and ripely sweet, and it's hard to keep from eating most of them. Once the seeds are out, the fleshy halves get spread out on a cookie sheet, one layer thick. After a while, my fingers get coated with the sticky rose hip goop, and I lick them a lot. I think how good a jam these would make, and maybe if there is enough, I'll try it. I pop the cookie sheet into the oven, and prop the door open for ventilation.

Hours later, the fruits are half the size they were earlier. They are less juicy, and darker, but still many of them feel fleshy so I put them back into the oven for a few more hours. The kitchen smells delicious. Even just the tiny bit of heat the oven makes fills the room with a sweet and spicy smell, and I walk through as often as I can, just for the fragrance.

Experiences with Rose Hips

Last year I used a handful of rose hips in a cough syrup of Solomon's seal and pine bark, and it gave the syrup a nice flavor. I figured the added vitamin C would be helpful in a cold or cough, and this year I'll try it again.

HORSETAIL
Equisetum species

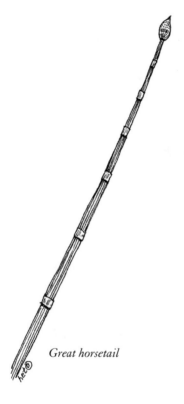

Great horsetail

Reflections: Beside the path stands a swampy area where tall, dead trees poke up here and there. The whole marsh is full of cattails going to seed, leaves brown and dry and bent. The cattail bases stand in water, and there are matted places where animals have made trails. I bend to see a patch of green that shows in the water, and find the weather-withered shoots of horsetail. Here, standing tall and thick, is the horsetail I went all the way to the ocean to see.

Description: Horsetail is believed to be one of the earliest plants on earth, and its survivors these days are similar in appearance, although much smaller in size. Two species of *Equisetum* are found in fair abundance in wet soil or near bodies of water, including drainage ditches. Both species are green and hollow and are usually dryish, even when freshly gathered, except for a bit of juice that exudes when picked. Either of the types can be used. Horsetail can attain 2 to 2¹/₂ feet in height.

Great horsetail or scouring rush grows as a single stalk, vertically ridged, with no projecting leaves or branches. Evenly spaced ridges along the stalk are marked with papery scales. Each single stalk is nonbranching.

Most commonly seen inland is the *Equisetum arvense,* known commonly as field horsetail. This has the same ridged single stem, but also has narrow, papery, leaflike projections that jut out from each joint in a whorled fashion, giving it the appearance of a horse's tail, or a tiny pine tree.

Medicinal Uses: The two species of horsetail act as a simple diuretic and astringent, which makes it suitable for lower urinary tract infections where it will increase easy flow of urine and help reduce inflammation of tissues. It can be used along with other herbs as a remedy for kidney stones. It is also hemostatic and can help stop bleeding in urinary tract infections or in heavy menses. Horsetail can also be used externally to help stop slow bleeding from minor wounds.

Field horsetail

Harvesting: Gather the stems or fertile shoots above ground, during their growing season, which is usually June through September. Bundle at the bases in small batches, and hang to dry. Horsetail dries fairly easily, and should be stored as soon as it is crumbly.

Dosages: To make a pleasant-tasting tea, use 1 tablespoon of the dried herb to 1 cup of boiling water three or four times daily. Steep 20 minutes. A fresh-plant tincture may also be made.

CAUTION: If used over a prolonged period of time or in very large amounts, horsetail can be irritating to intestinal mucosa and to tissues of the urinary tract.

This morning I walk down to Big Sandy to see the lake once more before the snows come. The morning is quiet and nice, overcast, with the sky full of clouds and a little blue showing through.

Yesterday deer season started, so the air was noisy with echoes of shots. Today, Sunday, there is no hunting and things are pretty still.

The air is cold but not bad. At the farm, cows stare and turn their heads to keep track of me. I walk down the hill thinking about the deer, about the special places down the development road where I know they congregate, and where now roads have been carved that hunters can drive into. I wish there were some way to interfere. I've thought about patrolling the woods, going out early every morning and late every day singing at the top of my lungs to warn the deer, but I probably won't. Yesterday I drove behind a hunter with a huge, bloody buck lying in the back of his open truck—a grisly sight. Today, walking into these woods, all I can do is wish the deer well and send quiet apologies for my species.

Along the roadside, most leaves have disappeared, and I can see into the woods deeper than before. Water gurgles in a stream that runs alongside the road, and in it, bright green moss still gleams on fallen logs. The air smells like balsam, and I take deep, long breaths, trying to fix the scent in my brain. At the bottom of the hill, I walk to the lake that stands behind a row of cottages. Here the soil is sandy, marked with tracks of a large deer, and I walk solidly over it, erasing evidence.

A narrow crescent beach lines the lake that is mirror smooth. Sun has just touched the water, and curls of golden mist lift and disappear. The lake is like glass, reflecting clouds and dark evergreens. In a little distance, tiny ripples of fish feeding disturb the surface. The ripples drift farther away, and the air on the water is colder. My toes get cold, too, so I get up to keep walking.

Next to the lake is a swampy area where cattails grow thick beside gray and weathered trees. The water is covered with dry, grayish grass that looks brittle, and I bend to see it close up. I trace one stalk to its base, and lift up a soggy sprig of horsetail.

The base is still lush and green and juicy, with ridges along its length and evenly spaced bracts. Farther up, the spike has shoots that have turned beige and papery with the cold. The farther I walk, the more horsetail I see. It forms the undergrowth in the wet places where cattail stands. The plants that grow protected under the giant cattail are green still, and I pick a huge armload to take home. When I turn to go, my toes are numb and freezing. I walk fast up the long steep hill, up through the woods to the back field and home.

Kitchen Notes

I bundle the horsetail to dry. It is funny stuff, so stiff and slippery it slides out of the strings that aren't tight enough. The pieces rustle against each other. They smell mostly wet and green, a lovely scent, and I decide to let them hang in the herb room even after they are dry.

Experiences with Horsetail

Just last week I used horsetail for a woman with a mild bladder infection. It went into a tea along with pyrola and pipsissewa, but would be fine to use all by itself. After a week of using horsetail, the woman reported no more symptoms from her infection, and now she will keep horsetail on hand for future use.

BURDOCK
Arctium lappa and *minor*

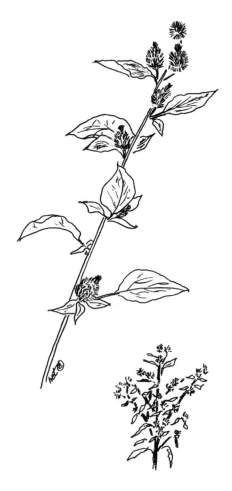

Reflections: I walk for a long time, eyes focused on the ground, looking for burdock root. The trail I follow leads through the beaten grass and then up a slight slope to the road. On a little rise, there is a den where some animal lives. Huge burdock leaves form a downy protective cover for the entrance, and bristly seeds cling to the grasses nearby.

Description: Burdock is a shrub-like plant commonly found in old fields, waste places, and disturbed soil. It seems to prefer soil that gets adequate moisture, and it is common in various regions of the country where soil has been disturbed.

The leaves vary in size, from basal leaves, which may be up to 18 inches in length and 8 inches wide, to smaller leaves at the top of the plant. The lower leaves have heart-shaped bases. First-year burdock plants occur as a basal cluster of leaves, while second-year plants have a central flower stem sprouting from lower leaves. Plant height is up to 5 feet in the common burdock and up to 9 feet in the great burdock.

Burdock flowers are bright purple and occur in bristly overlapping bracts with sharply hooked tips. Flower heads in the common burdock are up to 1 inch in length and up to 2 inches in length in the great burdock. Fruit forms from the same prickly head, and the sharp bracts stiffen, allowing the fruit to cling to anything it touches, thereby dispersing the dark seeds within.

Medicinal Uses: Burdock is known herbally as an alterative and blood purifier, and it is most commonly used in chronic skin conditions such as eczema and psoriasis, where it will help the body eliminate toxins and move toward a healthful systemic balance. Burdock root is somewhat diuretic and diaphoretic, and it is excreted by the kidneys and sweat glands, accounting for its usefulness in skin conditions. Burdock is also known as an herbal bitter, and as such, it stimulates the flow of bile and aids digestion. Burdock is useful in promoting overall health, especially when used in chronic, long-standing conditions.

Harvesting: Dig the first- or second-year roots in the late fall before the ground freezes. Check second-year plant roots (those that have produced flowers and seed burrs) thoroughly, since they are susceptible to rot, especially if growing in damp soil. Clean the roots well, slice into thin pieces, and dry on screens. The dried roots may be stored as they are, or they can be powdered in a blender to use in capsule form.

Dosages: For tea, place 1 tablespoon of dried root into 1 cup of cold water, bring to a boil on the stove, and simmer 15–20 minutes, covered. Strain, and drink 1 cup of tea two to three times daily. In capsule form, one capsule of powdered root can be taken three times daily. Burdock should be taken for at least 2 or 3 weeks before determining its usefulness.

I walk out to the back field to search for burdock. The sun is high in the sky, and a very little breeze blows. There are lots of beaten trails through the dry grass and I follow one that seems popular. It leads from the apple trees, across the field, and then splits off in several directions. There is coyote scat along the way, fresh and full of apple peels.

Back down behind the fruit trees, milkweed stands in large clumps, seeding. It is dry and gray, weathered looking, and brittle pods hold fluffs of seed silk that blow, shining, in the breeze. Next to the milkweed the huge, irregular, oblong leaves of first-year burdock spread flat along the ground. Each leaf has a long, thick stalk, but the plant bears no central stem.

I walk along the rocky knoll to a place where bouldery rocks make the going hard, and keep my eyes open for second-year plants. Suddenly, my sweater arm is full of sticky burrs that cling in clumps. I pick each one off carefully, and see behind me several tall, branched stalks with burrs clustered here and there. I decide to harvest a second-year root, put the shovel in a bit away from the dried stem, and hop on to it. But the ground is full of stones, and I don't get very far. Finally, I find a plant whose roots are not hiding underneath a boulder, and dig around it in a circle. The root I pull up is long and rough looking and knotted together with the root from a younger plant. The main root is covered with a dark layer of bark that peels away easily to expose a white inner core. Some of the branches of the root are soft and black, rotted, so I break these parts off and throw them away. The smaller roots come up easily, and are smooth with thinner bark, so I work on these. But every time I move, I get stuck again. The burrs from nearby plants have tucked themselves into the folds of my sweater, and around my ankles a ring of burrs clings to my socks. Every movement is uncomfortable.

Finally, I have a mixture of first- and second-year roots, and am ready to go. I walk down to the stream's edge where beavers toppled sapling trees for a dam this early summer. The water is high and dark with many days' rain. Burdock grows here, too, smaller plants creeping through the brush. I follow the animal trail home, and pick a few apples on the way.

Kitchen Notes

At home, the knotted roots get cleaned under running water. A few earthworms try to hide in the dark soil. I pop them out the back door onto the ground, and come back to clean more roots. On the cutting board, I start to slice the cleaned burdock. The small young roots slice easily, and have white flesh with an obvious dark outer layer. I taste a piece, expecting it to be bitter, but it's not. Actually, it's quite tasty, and I remember that burdock root can be eaten as a vegetable. There's no bad taste at all. I work on a large, older root, whose bark is darker, and whose length is furrowed a bit. I taste a piece of this root, and find it isn't bad either. I'm beginning to think there's something wrong with these roots. I thought burdock was supposed to be bitter, but these roots taste fine. I'll have to try gathering some in another place to see if soil makes a difference. Or maybe wait until there's a dry spell. These roots were gathered after several days of rain, and the soil was heavy and damp. Maybe that made a difference.

In just the time it takes to finish the work, the root slices become darker. It will be a week or so before they're ready to store. In the meantime, I'll probably gather more, to see if soil does make a differ-ence. So much to learn! But that's what I love about herbs—there are always surprises!

HAWTHORN BERRIES
Crataegus species

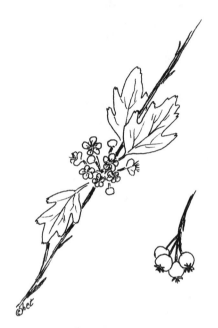

Reflections: In the herb room, the season is winding down. There is motherwort to cut and put away, and a handful of cleavers. There is still horsetail to process, and burdock gathered just last week is almost dry. In a basket, hawthorn berries nest. They are bright and scarlet, the only true color in this backdrop of dried plants. I stir them with my fingers and pick one to eat.

Description: There are over fifty species of *Crataegus* that grow in the Northeast, and the most common bear white flowers and have sharp spines along their branches. They are generally woody shrubs or small trees that bear edible fruit that looks somewhat like a rose hip. The hawthorns are attractive plants and are often planted as ornamentals.

The official species of traditional medicinal use is *Crataegus oxyacantha,* although any of the species may be used. Identification of the various species is difficult, a botanical reference should be used if this is desired. In general, the species may be used interchangeably.

Leaves of the hawthorns are alternate and irregularly lobed. The blossoms are white to pinkish white, with five petals. Fruit occurs as a bright, shiny, scarlet berry, although in some species may be yellowish. The height of the plants ranges from 3 to 30 feet. In many regions, jams and jellies are made of the fruit, which is often too astringent to be eaten without such preparation.

Medicinal Uses: Hawthorn berries have been used traditionally as a heart tonic. They are considered tonic and hypotensive in action and work gently without any toxicity or cumulative effect. Hawthorn is useful in heart problems generally, where it will help to normalize heart action without putting strain on the vascular system. It is also said to be helpful in hypertension, where it acts as a tonic to the heart and circulatory system, and may help to prevent or diminish arteriosclerosis. Specifically, hawthorn is a helpful adjunct to be used in heart weakness or heart failure and in mitral valve insufficiency. It can be used in angina as well.

Harvesting: Gather the ripe berries in fall, when full and colorful. Dry by spreading out on baskets or screens, being sure they are well aerated. To prevent spoilage, dry out of the sun. Berries may also be placed one layer thick on a cookie sheet, and dried in an oven set at its lowest temperature for several hours. A tincture can be made from fresh berries shortly after harvesting or from the dried berries at any time.

Dosage: For tea, cover spoons of the dried berries with boiling water in a cup, and allow to steep for 15–20 minutes. The tea can be drunk three times daily over a long period of time. For the tincture, take 10–30 drops three times daily.

FROM THE AUTHOR'S JOURNAL
NOVEMBER 12

It's another nice day. Sun steals over the treetops in the eastern sky and paints the morning bright. Already I have heard gunshots, early hunters, but the day is mostly quiet. Blue jays in the sumacs dive down for seed on the dooryard stair railing, and burst into flight again with a flutter of wings when they discover me.

I am out for a walk to look for any signs of green along the roadsides. This year I seem to be clinging to the time before snows come. Down Porter Road, there is lush green moss on logs and along the stone walls, but everything else has faded. The remains of fireweed hang over the little stream, tall skinny stems topped with brown curling leaves and a fluff of silky seed hairs that blow in a breeze. Where lady's slipper grew in clusters, there is no sign of them. Not one wide leaf, not one dried flower stalk has survived. Only the evergreens along the road stand full. Most other things are bare, and the forest floor is a cushion of dry, brown leaves that smell like winter coming.

At the entrance to a little path, my eyes catch on something bright in the frail light of these woods, and I step into the brush to check it out. Hard, scarlet berries the size of small rose hips tip each woody branch of a little tree. The fruit is held in clusters. Some pieces look chewed up a bit, but most are solid and fresh, just coming into ripeness in the past few nights of cold.

Along the woody twigs, long pointed thorns stand out, and I decide this must be hawthorn—the first I've seen this season. Mostly, the leaves blend in with those of neighboring small trees, so the plant doesn't stand out until its fruit ripens and colors. Now that the berries are scarlet, they are ready to be harvested, so I fill two pockets with them.

I save a few out to eat, and split one open with a fingernail. The berry is mostly seed. Hard, brown, pointy seeds are nestled in the flesh, making up the bulk of the fruit. I peel away a section of the cream-colored flesh, and taste it, and am surprised. There is an instant burst of fruity taste almost like the citric flavor of rose hips. The taste is sharp at first, not bad at all, but when I keep chewing the taste turns pretty bland. The texture is okay, too, and I think hawthorn would be good survival food, something to eat if there were nothing else. I chew on another berry and imagine it doing good things for my heart.

By now the sun has leaked through these woods, letting me know that the day is getting on. I pack up the berries and leave for home.

Experiences with Hawthorn Berries

I've only used hawthorn a few times, mostly as a tonic for the heart, and for people with high blood pressure. Lately I've offered it to a friend's father who has undergone heart and artery surgery. We're hoping it will help tone the arteries and that he can forego further surgery. His latest report was positive.

Last year, I talked with a physician who had been working with a man affected by serious heart trouble. The man told his doctor that he felt he owed the past 10 years of his life to hawthorn—that without it he wouldn't be alive. A pretty amazing statement. It makes me want to try hawthorn even more. I stir the berries with my fingers, turning them over to dry better, and get on with chores.

BARBERRY
Berberis vulgaris and *thunbergii*

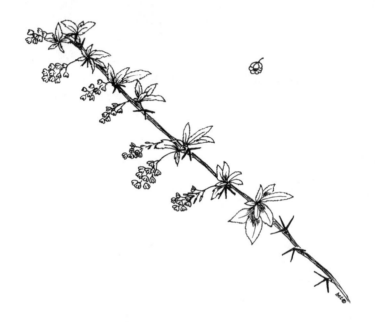

Reflections: I carry the barberry home gingerly, clutching the bright roots and dragging the bristly branches behind me. At home, I finally resort to using a chain saw to separate the roots from the stems, and accumulate enough barberry roots to use. I go in to clean and process the herb and catch sight of myself in a mirror. Hair full of brambly thorns and scraps of twigs, shirtfront a pattern of yellow blotches, face and hands covered with scratches—I look like a wild woman.

Description: The Barberry family is composed of spiny-stemmed shrubs common to meadows and thickets. Two barberry species are common to the Northeast, and they may be used interchangeably for medicinal purposes.

The common barberry, *Berberis vulgaris,* has leaves of varying length, from 1 to 3 inches long. The leaves are toothed and grow along the gray-barked stem in whorled clusters; the branches have sharp three-pronged spiny thorns. The roots are bright yellow in color, and the flowers are pale yellow. The blossoms are $1/4$ inch wide, with six petals. They occur in many-flowered racemes drooping from the leaf axils.

In the Japanese barberry, *Berberis thunbergii,* leaves are simple and have smooth margins. They occur in whorls along the stems. Flowers are the same yellow color, but they occur singly or in small loose clusters sprouting from leaf axils. The thorns in this species are single.

Fruit in both species is a bright scarlet, elliptical-shaped berry that matures in fall.

Medicinal Uses: Barberry root has a bitter taste and is commonly used as an herbal bitter to stimulate the digestive processes. Barberry is traditionally used as a liver herb and it is helpful in relieving any problems where sluggish liver functions are suspected. Barberry is a cholagogue, promoting the flow of bile. It is useful in chronic gallbladder disease or in the tendency to form gallstones.

Barberry is also antipyretic and anti-inflammatory and can be used to help reduce fevers. The root and root bark also have laxative properties and work gently to stimulate movement of the intestinal tract.

Harvesting: The roots of barberry should be dug in the fall after a frost or two. Clean and slice the roots thinly, or strip the root bark off if only the bark is to be used. Spread the root or root bark out on screens or other appropriate material. Store when completely dry. A tincture may be made of the root or the root bark, either fresh or dried. The dried plant parts may also be powdered for use in capsules.

Dosages: To make a tea, place 1 tablespoon of dried root or root bark into a pan, and cover with 1 cup of water. Bring to a boil, and simmer for 15–30 minutes on low heat. Strain out plant material, and drink three times a day. For the tincture, take 20–60 drops ($1/4$–$1/2$ teaspoon) three times a day. The powdered root or root bark can be taken in "00" capsules three times a day if desired.

I come out to harvest barberry before winter closes us in completely. In the backyard, six mourning doves are waddling about searching for seed. When I step out of the door, they take off with a burst of wings flapping, and make plaintive squeaking noises as they go. The air is dry and cool and getting colder, full of winter threatening. Sunrise is streaky scarlet, and now the flaming sun peeps over the ridge and gleams in windows.

Today there is barberry to do, one last herb to harvest before the ground freezes. I walk through the back field and down to the stone wall where barberry grows near the old apple trees. The hill slopes sharply down to the woods, and the field is divided by the stone wall laid maybe centuries ago when this land was first cleared. The fruit trees stand on either side of the wall, and growing almost from beneath the stones is barberry. It is full of bright berries that are shriveling with the recent cold. Tall branches make a great tangle that pokes up into the air like a threat. There are no leaves, but all the angled branches are covered with sharp thorns.

I walk around the prickly reaches of the plant, trying to decide where to start. In one place, the branches lean a bit, and there is room enough for me to stand close if I bend over. I plant the shovel in, dig for a while in the cold earth, and get nowhere. The main roots go much deeper than my shovel. I kneel to follow the root underground with my hands and end up scrabbling in a hole two feet deep, trying to catch as much root as I can. Thorny branches grab at me, tangling in my hair, and I move carefully, chipping off small lengths of rootlet with the spade. Finally, a large piece of root with its connected branches breaks away.

The barberry roots are brilliant yellow, impossible to get confused with those of any neighboring bushes. Where the shovel has nicked the root bark, yellow shows through bright and clear. I try cutting the gathered roots from their attached stems, and finally give up. I pat the earth back into place and stamp around on it. The remaining roots will put out new growth in the spring, so barberry can grow where is has for years. I make the trek back up the hill with the barberry, fighting the now-fierce wind.

Kitchen Notes

In the kitchen, the roots get scrubbed under cold water, and then cut into small bits. My hands grow yellow and taste bitter when I bring them to my mouth. Some of the barberry goes right away into a jar with alcohol, for tincture. Within seconds, the very yellow color seeps into the liquid. Then, because I've heard that root bark is best to use, I strip away as much of this as I can from the remaining roots, and cut it into small pieces. These get spread out to dry on a basket. This way, I can decide for myself whether there is much difference in potency between the whole root and the root bark. By the time I'm finished, the barberry tincture is a deep amber and gleams like a gem when I hold it up to the light.

Experiences with Barberry

Last year I used barberry as a tea. Recovering from a feverish flu, my digestive system was still limping along, and I used barberry as an herbal bitter and laxative. The taste was intensely bitter, and all I could manage was a few swallows before each meal. Oddly, though my mouth hated me for drinking the barberry tea, my body seemed to crave it, and I continued to take the tea for several days. After a while, my digestive system recovered, and I stopped the tea.

Outside now, the air is bitter cold. A solid sheet of gray masks the sky, and tiny, icy pellets assault the windows. Soon the air hisses with the sound of sleet hitting branches and pelting dry dead leaves, searing the ground. In the back field, the naked branches of barberry poke up, coated with a slick of ice that will protect them from the coming freezes. In the spring, I'll watch for barberry again, for its pretty yellow blossoms that come soon after the leaves. Then, the cycle will start all over again— for barberry, for the Earth and all her joyful gifts, and for me.

BIBLIOGRAPHY

Blumenthal, Mark et al. *The Complete German Commission E Report: Therapeutic Guide to Herbal Medicine,* 1998.

British Herbal Medical Association. *British Herbal Pharmacopoeia.* Lane House, Cowling, Nr. Keighley, West Yorks, 1979.

Christopher, Dr. John R. *School of Natural Healing.* Provo, Utah: Biworld Publishers, Inc., 1979.

Duke, James. *Herbs of the Bible: 2000 Years of Plant Medicine.* Loveland, Colorado: Interweave Press, 1999.

Felter, Harvey Wickes. *The Eclectic Materia Medic, Pharmacology and Therapeutics.* Ohio: John K. Scudder, 1922.

Foster, Steven. *Herbal Bounty! The Gentle Art of Herb Culture.* Layton, Utah: Peregrine Smith Books, 1984.

Foster, Steven, and Duke, James. *Medicinal Plants and Herbs of Eastern and Central North America* (Peterson Field Guides), 2nd edition. Boston: Houghton Mifflin Co., 2000.

Gibbons, Euell. *Stalking the Healthful Herbs.* Brattleboro, Vermont: Alan C. Hood, Inc., 1974.

Harrar, Sari. *The Woman's Book of Healing Herbs.* Emmaus, Pennsylvania: Rodale Press, Inc., 1999.

Hoffman, David. *The Holistic Herbal.* Findhorn, Moray, Scotland: The Findhorn Press, 1983.

Kloss, Jethro. *Back to Eden.* Loma Linda, California: Back to Eden Books, 1981.

Kowalchik, Claire and Hylton. *William H. Rodale's Illustrated Encyclopedia of Herbs*. Emmaus, Pennsylvania: Rodale Press, 1987.

Lad, Dr. Vasant, and David Frawley. *The Yoga of Herbs*. Sante Fe: Lotus Press, 1986.

Medical Economics Corporation, Inc. *Physician's Desk Reference for Herbal Medicine: Information Standard for Complementary Medicine*. Montvale, New Jersey, 1998.

Moerman, Daniel E. *Native American Ethnobotany*. Portland, Oregon: Timber Press, 1998.

Moore, Michael. *Medicinal Plants of the Mountain West*. Sante Fe: Museum of New Mexico Press, 1982.

Newcomb, Lawrence. *Newcomb's Wildflower Guide*. Boston, Toronto: Little, Brown, 1977.

Niering, William A., and Olmstead, Nancy C. *The Audubon Society Field Guide to North American Wildflowers*. New York: Alfred A. Knopf, 1984.

Soule, Deb. *A Woman's Book of Herbs*. Carol Publishing Group, Secaucus, New Jersey, 1998.

Tierra, Michael. *The Way of Herbs*. New York: Washington Square Press, 1983.

Weil, Andrew. *Health and Healing*. Boston: Houghton Mifflin Co., 1983.

HERBAL ASSOCIATIONS
AND SOCIETIES

AMERICAN BOTANICAL COUNCIL AND HERB RESEARCH FOUNDATION, "educating the public on the use of herbs and phytomedicines." Offers monthly educational journal *HerbalGram,* research and world news on herbal medicines, medicinal herb and drug interaction consultations, legal and regulatory information, ethnobotanical tours, educational activities and conferences, international product development information, herbal education packets, and numerous other services. Address: P.O. Box 144345, Austin, TX 78714-4345, (512) 926-4900.

AMERICAN HERB ASSOCIATION, offering quarterly publications, conference and workshop schedules, updates on recent research. Address: P.O. Box 353, Rescue, CA 95672.

AMERICAN HERBALIST GUILD, "revitalizing our herbal traditions." Offering quarterly publications, directory of professional members and herbal education, assistance to cooperation between herbalists and health care practitioners. Address: 1931 Gaddis Road, Canton, GA 30115, ahgoffice@earthlink.net, www.healthy.net\ herbalists, (770) 751-6021.

AVENA INSTITUTE, "deepening our connections to the natural world." Offers educational workshops with herbalist Deb Soule, herbal products including alcohol- and glycerin- based tinctures, conferences, and apprenticeships. Address: P.O. Box 333, West Rockport, ME 04865, (207) 594-0694.

United Plant Savers, "a nonprofit education corporation dedicated to preserving native medicinal plants." Offers a quarterly newsletter, medicinal plant information and occasional free plant give-aways to members, botanical sanctuary in Ohio, directory of nursery stock of native and endangered medicinal plants, updated lists of at-risk plants in various areas of the country, slide show available for rental, land consultation service, and a conference and workshop calendar. Address: P.O. Box 98, East Barre, VT 05649, (802) 496-7053, info@plantsavers.org.

Numerous other herbal organizations exist. Check with one of the above-listed for groups in your area.

GLOSSARY

ABORTIFACIENT: A substance that may cause miscarriage.

ALTERATIVE: A substance that, when taken over a period of time in the presence of long-standing illness, will gradually move the body systems toward a normal balance.

ANALGESIC: A substance that relieves pain.

ANTHELMINTIC: A substance that can help to destroy and expel intestinal parasites. (See also *vermifuge.*)

ANTIBIOTIC: Acting to destroy or inhibit the growth of microorganisms.

ANTI-INFLAMMATORY: Acting to reduce inflammation and associated symptoms such as pain, swelling, and so on.

ANTINEOPLASTIC: Acting to arrest the growth of abnormal or cancerous cells.

ANTIPYRETIC: Acting to reduce a fever.

ANTISEPTIC: Acting to destroy or slow the growth of bacteria.

ANTISPASMODIC: Acting to relieve or prevent spasms of muscles and associated tissues.

ANTITUSSIVE: Acting to reduce or relieve coughs.

AROMATIC: A substance containing volatile oils that have a strong and stimulating scent.

ASTRINGENT: Acting to constrict tissues and, in the process, reduce the release of fluids such as blood, secretions, and so forth.

BITTER TONIC: An herb or group of herbs that stimulate the digestive processes.

BLOOD PURIFIER: An herb that stimulates the digestive and excretory processes of the body to aid in the elimination of waste products.

CARDIAC TONIC: A substance that enhances function of the heart while not directly working on the heart muscle.

CARDIOACTIVE: A substance that acts directly on the muscles of the heart.

CARMINATIVE: Acting to relieve or expel intestinal gas and associated cramping.

CATHARTIC: A substance that causes rapid intestinal purging.

CHOLAGOGUE: Promotes the flow of bile.

DECONGESTANT: A substance that acts to break up congestion.

DEMULCENT: A substance that is soothing to mucous membranes.

DIAPHORETIC: Acting to stimulate sweating.

DISINFECTANT: A substance that is antiseptic.

DIURETIC: A substance that acts to increase the flow of urine.

EMETIC: Acting to produce vomiting.

EMMENAGOGUE: A substance that promotes and regulates menstrual functions.

EMOLLIENT: A substance that is soothing and protective to the skin.

EXPECTORANT: A substance that promotes the flow of mucus from the lungs, bronchi, and throat.

FEBRIFUGE: A substance that acts to reduce fever.

HEMOSTATIC: Acting to stop bleeding.

HEPATIC: A substance that acts on the liver.

HYPNOTIC: A substance that induces sleep.

HYPOGLYCEMIA: A condition of low blood sugar.

HYPOTENSIVE: Acting to lower blood pressure.

LAXATIVE: A substance that acts to tone and promote bowel movement.

LYMPHATIC TONIC: A substance that acts to tone and promote proper function of the lymph system and associated organs such as the lymph nodes, spleen, liver, and thymus.

MUCILAGINOUS: A thick, slippery consistency.

MUSCLE RELAXANT: A substance that acts to relax voluntary and involuntary muscles.

NERVINE: A substance that has a soothing and quieting effect on the nervous system.

PARTURIENT: A substance that aids in preparing the body for childbirth.

PURGATIVE: A substance that promotes thorough cleansing of the intestines.

SALICIN: An aspirin-like compound used to relieve pain and reduce inflammation.

SEDATIVE: Acting to soothe nerves and promote sleep.

STIMULANT: Acting to excite or hasten a process.

TONIC: Acting to tone and strengthen a particular system or the body in general.

VERMIFUGE: A substance that acts to kill and/or expel intestinal parasites.

VULNERARY: Acting to heal wounds.

INDEX

A

Acne, 203, 205, 207, 210

Alcohol, 16–17, 18–19

Allergies, 26, 53

Alteratives: burdock, 233; chickweed, 65; cleavers, 57; red clover, 80; violet, 45

Analgesics: mint, 147; shinleaf, 61; wintergreen, 30

Anodynes: wild lettuce, 175; witch hazel, 207

Anorexia, 194

Anti-inflammatories: barberry, 241; boneset, 151; chickweed, 65; cleavers, 57; gentian, 194; plantain, 72; shinleaf, 61; St. John's-wort, 122; willow, 25–28; yarrow, 76

Anti-neoplastics: violet, 45

Antipyretics: barberry, 241; yarrow, 76

Antiseptics: hops, 188; juniper, 184; pipsissewa, 114; shinleaf, 61; violet, 45; white pine, 41; willow, 26; wintergreen, 30; yarrow, 76

Antispasmodics: blue cohosh, 138; blue vervain, 159; boneset, 151; catnip, 33–36; coltsfoot, 163; lobelia, 130; mint, 147; motherwort, 155; red clover, 80; skunk cabbage, 212; St. John's-wort, 122; sundew, 106; valerian, 142; wild cherry, 179

Antitussives: red clover, 80; wild cherry, 179

Antivirals: St. John's-wort, 122

Anxiety, 122, 142, 147, 159, 161, 190

Aromatics: Mint, 147

Arthritis, 26, 30, 65, 151, 175, 184, 185, 194

Asthma, 41, 72–73, 85, 98, 106, 130, 132, 163, 165, 212

Astringents: bayberry, 217; blackberry, 167; blueberry, 118; comfrey, 84; hops, 188; horsetail, 229; mullein, 98; partridgeberry, 94; plantain, 72; raspberry, 102; rose hips, 225; self-heal, 126; shepherd's purse, 110; shinleaf, 61; St. John's-wort, 122; sweet fern, 90; wintergreen, 30; witch hazel, 207

Athlete's foot, 171

B

Barberry (*Berberis* species), 240–44

Bayberry (*Myrica* species), 216–19

Bed-wetting, 98

Blackberry *(Rubus allegheniensis)*, 166–69

Bladder control, 98

Bladder infections, 30, 57, 61, 76, 78, 114, 116, 118, 122, 163, 184, 186, 229, 231

Bleeding, 94, 102, 110, 229

Blood pressure, elevated, 223, 237, 239

Blood purifiers, 203, 233

Blueberry (*Vaccinium* species), 117–20

Blue cohosh *(Caulophyllum thalictroides)*, 137–40

Blue vervain *(Verbena hastata)*, 158–61

Boneset *(Eupatorium perfoliatum)*, 150–53

Bronchitis, 41, 45, 72–73, 85, 98, 106, 130, 163, 179, 212

Bruises, 122, 126

Bug bites. *See* Insect bites

Burdock (*Arctium* species), 232–35

Burns, 57, 85, 88, 122, 207

C

Cancer, 45, 80

Carminatives: catnip, 33–36; juniper, 184;

mint, 147; yarrow, 76

Catnip *(Nepeta cataria)*, 33–36

Checkerberry. *See* Wintergreen

Chicken pox, 114

Chickweed *(Stellaria media)*, 64–67

Childbirth, 102, 104, 110, 111, 138, 140; *see also* Pregnancy

Cholagogues: barberry, 241; dandelion, 221; greater celandine, 49; yellow dock, 203

Cleavers *(Galium aparine)*, 56–59

Colds, 26, 45, 53, 55, 76, 98, 126, 147, 149, 151, 153, 163, 212, 217, 225

Cold sores, 38

Colic, 34, 36, 134

Colitis, 188, 217

Coltsfoot *(Tussilago farfara)*, 162–65

Comfrey *(Symphytum officinale)*, 83–88

Congestion, 41, 43, 45, 80, 98, 198–99, 201

Constipation, 203, 205, 221

Coughs, 41, 43, 45, 72–73, 80, 82, 85, 106, 130, 132, 163, 165, 179, 182, 212, 227

Curly dock. *See* Yellow dock

D

Dandelion *(Taraxacum officinale)*, 220–23

Decoction, 15–16

Demulcents: coltsfoot, 163; comfrey, 84; mullein, 98; plantain, 72–73; Solomon's seal, 198–99; sundew, 106

Depression, 122

Diabetes, 118, 120, 221, 223

Diaper rash, 72

Diaphoretics: bayberry, 217; blue vervain, 159; boneset, 151; burdock, 233; catnip, 33–36; elderberry, 53; mint, 147; skunk cabbage, 212; yarrow, 76

Diarrhea, 72, 73, 90, 102–3, 110, 126, 167, 207, 208, 225

Digestive problems, 38, 134, 151, 184, 188, 194, 203, 233, 241, 243–44

Disinfectants: pipsissewa, 114

Diuretics: blueberry, 118; boneset, 151; burdock, 233; chickweed, 65; cleavers, 57; dandelion, 221; horsetail, 229; juniper, 184; mullein, 98; pipsissewa, 114; shepherd's

purse, 110; shinleaf, 61; St. John's-wort, 122; wintergreen, 30; yarrow, 76

Duodenal ulcers, 84

Dysentery, 167

E

Earaches, 98

Eczema, 45, 80, 203, 205, 221, 233

Edema, 57, 110, 223

Elderberry *(Sambucus species)*, 52–55

Emmenagogues: blue cohosh, 138; motherwort, 155; partridgeberry, 94; tansy, 134; yarrow, 76

Endometritis, 138

Expectorants: coltsfoot, 163; comfrey, 85; lobelia, 130; mullein, 98; plantain, 72–73; red clover, 80; skunk cabbage, 212; Solomon's seal, 198–99; sundew, 106; violet, 45; white pine, 41; wild cherry, 179; yarrow, 76

Eyestrain, 207, 208, 225

F

Fevers, 34, 36, 53, 55, 65, 126, 147, 149, 151, 153, 159, 194, 212, 217, 241

Fluid retention, 221

Flus, 26, 53, 55, 76, 78, 147, 149, 151, 153, 212, 225

Fungicides: jewelweed, 171

G

Gallbladder ailments, 49, 203, 221, 241

Gallstones, 49, 221, 241

Gentian *(Gentiana species)*, 193–96

Glycerin, 17, 20

Goldthread *(Coptis trifolia)*, 37–39

Gout, 118

Greater celandine *(Chelidonium majus)*, 48–51

Gum inflammations, 90, 126, 217

H

Hawthorn *(Crataegus species)*, 236–39

Hay fever, 26, 53

Headaches, 26, 142